Management of the Cleft Patient

Editor

KEVIN S. SMITH

ORAL AND MAXILLOFACIAL SURGERY CLINICS OF NORTH AMERICA

www.oralmaxsurgery.theclinics.com

Consulting Editor
RICHARD H. HAUG

May 2016 • Volume 28 • Number 2

ELSEVIER

1600 John F. Kennedy Boulevard • Suite 1800 • Philadelphia, Pennsylvania, 19103-2899

http://www.oralmaxsurgery.theclinics.com

ORAL AND MAXILLOFACIAL SURGERY CLINICS OF NORTH AMERICA Volume 28, Number 2
May 2016 ISSN 1042-3699, ISBN-13: 978-0-323-44477-4

Editor: John Vassallo; j.vassallo@elsevier.com
Developmental Editor: Colleen Viola

Oral and Maxillofacial Surgery Clinics of North America (ISSN 1042-3699) is published quarterly by Elsevier Inc., 360 Park Avenue South, New York, NY 10010-1710. Months of issue are February, May, August, and November. Business and Editorial Offices: 1600 John F. Kennedy Blvd., Suite 1800, Philadelphia, PA 19103-2899. Periodicals postage paid at New York, NY and additional mailing offices. Subscription prices are $385.00 per year for US individuals, $628.00 per year for US institutions, $100.00 per year for US students and residents, $455.00 per year for Canadian individuals, $753.00 per year for Canadian institutions, $520.00 per year for international individuals, $753.00 per year for international institutions and $235.00 per year for Canadian and foreign students/residents. To receive student/resident rate, orders must be accompanied by name or affiliated institution, date of term, and the *signature* of program/residency coordinator on institution letterhead. Orders will be billed at individual rate until proof of status is received. Foreign air speed delivery is included in all *Clinics* subscription prices. All prices are subject to change without notice. **POSTMASTER:** Send address changes to *Oral and Maxillofacial Surgery Clinics of North America,* Elsevier Periodicals **Customer Service, 11830 Westline Industrial Drive, St. Louis, MO 63146. Tel: 1-800-654-2452 (U.S. and Canada); 314-447-8871 (outside U.S. and Canada). Fax: 314-447-8029. E-mail: journals customerservice-usa@elsevier.com (for print support); journalsonlinesupport-usa@elsevier.com (for online support).**

Reprints. For copies of 100 or more, of articles in this publication, please contact the Commercial Reprints Department, Elsevier Inc., 360 Park Avenue South, New York, NY 10010-1710. Tel.: 212-633-3874; Fax: 212-633-3820; Email: reprints@elsevier.com.

Oral and Maxillofacial Surgery Clinics of North America is covered in *MEDLINE/PubMed (Index Medicus), Science Citation Index Expanded (SciSearch®), Journal Citation Reports/Science Edition*, and *Current Contents®/Clinical Medicine.*

Contributors

CONSULTING EDITOR

RICHARD H. HAUG, DDS
Professor and Chief, Oral Maxillofacial Surgery,
Carolinas Medical Center, Charlotte, North
Carolina

EDITOR

KEVIN S. SMITH, DDS
Clinical Professor and Residency Program
Director, Co-Director, The University of
Oklahoma, JW Keys Cleft and Craniofacial
Clinic, Co-Director, The University of Tulsa, MK
Chapman Cleft and Craniofacial Clinic,
Department of Oral and Maxillofacial Surgery,
The University of Oklahoma Health Sciences
Center, Oklahoma City, Oklahoma

AUTHORS

WAYNE BERRYHILL, MD
Oklahoma Otolaryngology Associates,
Norman, Oklahoma

CARLOS CRUZ, DDS
Medical Director of Cleft Craniofacial Team
at Valley Baptist Medical Center, Oral &
Craniofacial Center, PLLC, Edinburg, Texas

ANGELO CUZALINA, MD, DDS
Fellowship Director, Private Practice Tulsa
Surgical Arts, Tulsa, Oklahoma

RANDOLPH DEAL, PhD
Professor, University of Oklahoma Health
Sciences Center, Oklahoma City, Oklahoma

DAVID G. GAILEY, DDS
Consultant Surgeon, Providence Sacred Heart
Medical Center, Maxillofacial Cleft Team; Oral
and Maxillofacial Surgeon, Inland Oral Surgery,
Spokane, Washington

ROBERT S. GLADE, MD, FAAP
Volunteer Professor, Oromaxillofacial Surgery,
Oklahoma University, Oklahoma City,
Oklahoma; Adjunct Professor,
Otolaryngology–Head and Neck Surgery,
Oklahoma State University, Tulsa,
Oklahoma

BYRON T. HENRY, DDS
Free to Smile Foundation, President and
Founder, Columbus, Ohio; Cleft and
Craniofacial Surgical Fellow, University of
Oklahoma, Oklahoma City, Oklahoma

JEFFREY N. JAMES, MD, DDS
Assistant Professor, Department of Oral and
Maxillofacial Surgery, Louisiana State
University Health Science Center, New
Orleans, Louisiana; Team Surgeon, Cleft and
Craniofacial Team, New Orleans Children's
Hospital, New Orleans, Louisiana; Staff
Surgeon, 59th Medical Wing, Dental Training
Squadron, Lackland Air Force Base, San
Antonio, Texas; Private Practice, The Cleft and
Facial Cosmetic Surgery Center, Metairie,
Louisiana

CALVIN JUNG, MD, DDS
Private Practice, Premier Surgical Arts,
Houston, Texas

JEFFREY J. MOSES, DDS, FAACS
President/Founder, Smiles International
Foundation (SIF), Oklahoma City,
Oklahoma

WHITNEY J. ROCHELLE, DDS
PGY-2 Resident, Department of Oral and
Maxillofacial Surgery, University of Oklahoma
Health Sciences Center, Oklahoma City,
Oklahoma

DANIEL W. SCHLIEDER, MD, DDS
Resident Physician, Department of Oral and
Maxillofacial Surgery, Louisiana State

University Health Science Center, New
Orleans, Louisiana

MICHELLE A. SCOTT, DDS, MBA
Director of Orthodontic treatment program,
Nationwide Children's Hospital, Columbus,
Ohio, USA

KEVIN S. SMITH, DDS
Clinical Professor and Residency Program
Director, Co-Director, The University of
Oklahoma, JW Keys Cleft and Craniofacial
Clinic, Co-Director, The University of Tulsa, MK
Chapman Cleft and Craniofacial Clinic,
Department of Oral and Maxillofacial Surgery,
The University of Oklahoma Health Sciences
Center, Oklahoma City, Oklahoma

Contents

 Video content accompanies this article at http://www.oralmaxsurgery. theclinics.com

A multidisciplinary team is the standard of care and the cornerstone of management of cleft patients. With readily improving advanced diagnostic modalities, early prenatal diagnosis of cleft lip and palate increasingly becomes a topic of importance for both the team caring for and families of cleft patients. Maternal-fetal medicine is a fellowship subspecialty of obstetrics that can offer high-quality care and coordination to the cleft team. Both 3-D and 4-D sonography lead to early prenatal diagnosis of cleft patients; however, differences in training result in variations in its diagnostic accuracy.

Cleft lip and palate malformations affect the ability of infants to adequately feed. Choosing the appropriate feeding technique must allow functioning of the suck-swallow-breathing mechanism and development of oral-motor function. Feeding in the postsurgical setting should be returned to normal as soon as possible to maintain adequate nutritional intake and good wound healing, an essential component to cleft repair. This article outlines the complex mechanism of wound healing, gives options to augment the process of aesthetic scar healing, and presents feeding modifications.

The Latham appliance is an active presurgical orthopedic device used for cleft defects. Its long-term effects are debated. It was introduced to help surgeons achieve a more predictable surgical outcome; hence, it should be evaluated for its presurgical benefits. The device has been successful in expanding and aligning the maxillary segments; retruding protruded premaxillae; aligning bilateral alveolar ridges; placing less tension on surgical closures; and reducing fistulation rates. However, it has not been shown to have either a positive or negative long-term effect on maxillary development or occlusion. It is a valuable preoperative tool for surgeons treating cleft defects.

Over the last decade, presurgical orthopedic molding for the patient with cleft lip and palate has become much more common; it is even reasonable to assume it may be

this article have valuable contacts with local dentists and surgeons within the community. They also have insight into the local facilities, hospitals, water sources, sanitation conditions, and equipment potential.

ORAL AND MAXILLOFACIAL SURGERY CLINICS OF NORTH AMERICA

THE CLINICS ARE NOW AVAILABLE ONLINE!
Access your subscription at:
www.theclinics.com

Preface

The Esoteric but Essential Concerns of Treating Children with Cleft Lip and Palate

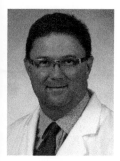

Kevin S. Smith, DDS
Editor

The title of this preface may be confusing for some not involved in the treatment of children with cleft lip and palate and other craniofacial disorders. However, in order for surgeons of any specialty to be intimately involved with treating children with cleft lip and palate, we must understand all of the related areas of concern regarding cleft lip and palate.

In this issue of *Oral and Maxillofacial Surgery Clinics of North America*, we attempted to address some major issues associated with cleft lip and palate. The surgeon entering the care of patients with cleft lip and palate and perhaps not originally trained to treat these children needs to understand the aspects of prenatal diagnosis, feeding, post-operative care, and speech issues caused by cleft palate, including diagnosis and treatment, audiologic issues, secondary rhinoplasties, and the truly difficult part of treating children with cleft lip and palate—funding for patients who have inadequate insurance coverage.

There have been several issues of *Oral and Maxillofacial Surgery Clinics of North America* prior to this one that addressed the technical aspects of cleft lip and palate closure, but in this issue, we truly focused our attention on some of the more vague aspects of patients with cleft lip and palate.

Kevin S. Smith, DDS
The University of Oklahoma
JW Keys Cleft and Craniofacial Clinic
The University of Tulsa
MK Chapman Cleft and Craniofacial Clinic
Department of Oral and Maxillofacial Surgery
The University of Oklahoma Health Sciences Center
1000 North Lincoln Boulevard, Suite 2000
Oklahoma City, OK 73104, USA

E-mail address:
kevin-smith@ouhsc.edu

Oral Maxillofacial Surg Clin N Am 28 (2016) ix
http://dx.doi.org/10.1016/j.coms.2016.03.001
1042-3699/16/$ – see front matter © 2016 Published by Elsevier Inc.

Prenatal Counseling, Ultrasound Diagnosis, and the Role of Maternal-Fetal Medicine of the Cleft Lip and Palate Patient

Jeffrey N. James, MD, DDS[a,b,c,d,*],
Daniel W. Schlieder, MD, DDS[a]

KEYWORDS

- Cleft • Congenital facial anomalies • Prenatal diagnosis • Maternal fetal medicine
- 3D/ 4D ultrasonography

KEY POINTS

- A multidisciplinary team is the standard of care and the cornerstone of management of cleft patients.
- With readily improving advanced diagnostic modalities, early prenatal diagnosis of cleft lip and palate increasingly becomes a topic of importance for both the team caring for and families of cleft patients.
- Maternal-fetal medicine (MFM) is a fellowship subspecialty of obstetrics that can offer high-quality care and coordination to the cleft team.
- Both 3-D and 4-D sonography lead to early prenatal diagnosis of cleft patients; however, differences in training result in variations in its diagnostic accuracy.

 Video content accompanies this article at http://www.oralmaxsurgery.theclinics.com

INTRODUCTION

Cleft lip, with or without cleft palate, is the most common congenital facial malformation, with a prevalence ranging from 1 in 500 to 1 in 2500 live births, depending on geographic origin and ethnic background.[1–3] With technologic advances, prenatal diagnostic modalities continue to improve, and it is now possible to diagnose craniofacial malformations well before birth. Thus, consideration must be given to the role these modalities have in regard to this unique patient population. A multidisciplinary team approach is now widely accepted as the standard of care in dealing with these complex patients. The role of the MFM physician and the importance of prenatal counseling continue to evolve with changing diagnostic approaches. By understanding this multidisciplinary, multimodality prenatal approach to cleft lip and palate patients, oral and maxillofacial surgeons are uniquely positioned to coordinate the complex treatment these patients require.

[a] Department of Oral and Maxillofacial Surgery, Louisiana State University Health Science Center, 1100 Florida Avenue, New Orleans, LA 70119, USA; [b] Cleft and Craniofacial Team, New Orleans Children's Hospital, 200 Henry Clay Avenue, New Orleans, LA 70118, USA; [c] 59th Medical Wing, Dental Training Squadron, Lackland Air Force Base, San Antonio, TX, USA; [d] The Cleft and Facial Cosmetic Surgery Center, 4420 Conlin, Suite #203, Metairie, LA 70006, USA
* Corresponding author. 4420 Conlin st, Suite 203, Metairie, LA 70006.
E-mail address: jnj39811@icloud.com; *Website:* https://cfcnola.com/us/

Oral Maxillofacial Surg Clin N Am 28 (2016) 145–151
http://dx.doi.org/10.1016/j.coms.2015.12.005

THE MULTIDISCIPLINARY TEAM

A well-coordinated interdisciplinary team has become the standard of care for the treatment of cleft lip and palate. Although various team approaches had been in place for more than 60 years, for a time there was no comprehensive statement on what a cleft/craniofacial team should look like. Work began in 1991 when the surgeon general issued a report on special needs children. Recognizing that children with craniofacial birth defects, including cleft lip and palate, were among those children with special health care needs, the Maternal and Child Health Bureau provided funding to the American Cleft Palate-Craniofacial Association (ACPA) for the purpose of identifying recommended practices in the care of patients with craniofacial anomalies.[4]

In 1998, the ACPA standards committee led by Dr Ronald Strauss conducted the first comprehensive national survey of the structure, function, and composition of cleft palate and craniofacial teams in the United States and Canada. Their findings from the survey noted discrepancies regarding the structure, distribution, regionalization, and resource allocation for cleft/craniofacial teams.[5] A dedicated effort was thus put under way by the ACPA and today their Commission on Approval of Teams has set forth guidelines on the standard cleft and craniofacial team composition. To be approved by the ACPA, a cleft team is required to include a designated patient care coordinator, speech-language pathologist, and orthodontic specialist as well as a surgeon, most commonly of oral and maxillofacial or plastic surgery background. Furthermore the team should provide access to adjunct professionals in the disciplines of pediatric dentistry, otolaryngology, pediatrics/primary care, genetics, audiology, and social work and psychology.[6] Further standards in addition to those for the cleft team are in place to be designated as a craniofacial team.

The comprehensive management of cleft lip and palate patients demands consideration of the complex anatomic deformity, psychosocial development, and the delicate balance between surgical repair and optimization of growth. The difficult nature of these issues are due to the iatrogenic effects of surgery on patient growth that often are directly complicating patients' psychosocial maturation as they move through speech development, enter school age, and continue through adolescence. From a surgical standpoint, the goals of successful management of cleft patients include

- Restoration of an acceptably esthetic lip, nose, and facial profile
- Closure of palatal defects
- Restoration of alveolar continuity
- Appropriate speech and language development
- Adequate oral hygiene and dental and periodontal health
- An appropriate jaw relationship that is conducive to masticatory function
- A smooth transition into social circles and school

To achieve these goals, a coordinated multidisciplinary team approach from birth through adolescence is critical to achieving success. A genetic analysis is warranted whenever a syndrome is suspected along with the anatomic craniofacial defect. An otolaryngology evaluation for eustachian tube and middle ear defects as well as audiology evaluation for hearing deficit is appropriate. A speech pathologist works closely with the patient from the time of speech development until well after the completion of palatal cleft repairs. A social worker has a valuable role to play because often these patient populations come from homes that are poorly equipped to deal with the unique challenges they present, from obtaining specialized feeding equipment to overcoming the financial hurdles these families may be faced with. Unfortunately, many of these children struggle with depression and anxiety issues that develop as they navigate the maze of social development and peer interactions, and a child psychiatrist is often a beneficial contributor in their care team. To better prepare a patient's family for the long road ahead of them, the role of prenatal counseling has become a cornerstone of the initial decision-making timing not only for how to best treat the patient but also to inform the family of what is to come. Although not specifically noted by the ACPA in their standard team composition guidelines, a newer subspecialty of obstetrics, the MFM physician, is well poised to provide accurate and timely prenatal diagnosis and counseling to these families.

NEED FOR PRENATAL COUNSELING

Much research has been done on the need for prenatal counseling. When parents discover a cleft malformation at birth, they often experience what is classified as a psychosocial crisis that is characterized by disappointment, helplessness, and desperation, which may lead to a period of severe emotional crisis for the parents. Often the parents feel guilty about the malformation and are concerned about the future of their child.[7] This emotional response can be mitigated by proper prenatal diagnosis, education, and planning. A recent survey conducted in Switzerland looked at how the parents of cleft patients viewed their experience with their prenatal consultations. The results of the study found the parents often used multiple sources of information—the obstetrician, the counsel by the cleft team surgeon, the parent support groups, and the Internet: 93% of the parents felt well prepared psychologically for the birth of their child and concerning the practical aspects of care; 54% felt relieved that their child was less affected than imagined; and 96% considered prenatal diagnosis a benefit.[8]

There is currently no appropriate intrauterine treatment of cleft lip and palate. Despite this, research has indicated that both mother and child benefit from early diagnosis and counseling. Rather than deal with the shock the diagnosis is bound to bring during the tumultuous aftermath of birth, the parents are able to spend time coming to terms with the reality of the malformation as well as have an appropriate amount of time in which to educate themselves about what the diagnosis means. Historically, the question arose whether early diagnosis of cleft lip or palate would lead to an increased rate of pregnancy termination. Some studies have shown that up to 10% of families consider pregnancy termination after they receive their prenatal diagnosis.[9] These scenarios have been discussed by medical ethicists for decades and the overwhelming body of evidence suggests that when adequate information is presented to the parents and they are given sufficient emotional support, they are able to see the excellent treatment options available to them and quickly resume their excitement for the upcoming birth.[10–12] Once an ultrasonographer discovers the facial cleft, the parents are then directed to the multidisciplinary care team for further action. The question no longer is, "Should we tell the parent?" but rather, "How is the best way to tell the parent?"

Most surveys also indicate that parents prefer to know the diagnosis prenatally. With this in mind, the question arises of who is the best person to initially deliver the diagnosis and who is best suited to continue the counseling in the weeks to follow. A study from Sweden looked at a total of 160 patients with cleft lip or palate or isolated cleft palate who were referred to one of the countries dedicated cleft centers. After exclusion of the isolated cleft palate patients, 38/40 children were diagnosed prenatally and 56/58 patients were diagnosed postnatally. In cases of a prenatal diagnosis, a majority (50%) were informed by the ultrasonographer. For the postnatal group (74%), diagnosis was routinely made by the delivery unit. In the prenatal group, most (78%) gave the information received during the prenatal counseling the highest mark, whereas only a third pointed to the ultrasound unit as having delivered the best information regarding the diagnosis. In the postnatal group, 20% gave the information received in the delivery unit the highest mark, whereas a majority of parents in the postnatal group gave the cleft team's information the highest mark.[13] The conclusion is obvious that the most accurate and soothing information comes once parents have been seen by a dedicated cleft provider, most commonly a cleft surgeon.

At the University of Oklahoma, the experience is similar. Smith and colleagues conducted surveys to compare the emotions experienced by those parents who were counseled prenatally versus those who received their initial counseling postnatally (Smith K, unpublished data, 2008). The prenatal group also had a follow-up survey after birth. The findings from their study are in **Figs. 1** and **2**,

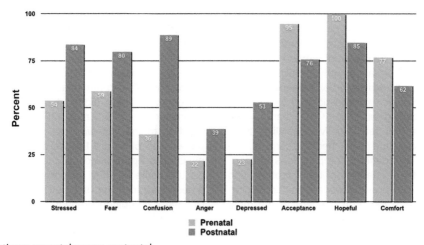

Fig. 1. Emotions: prenatal versus postnatal.

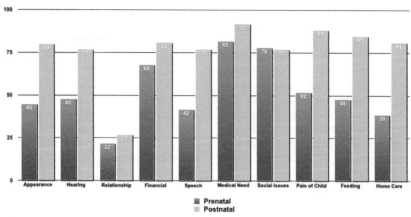

Fig. 2. Area of concern: prenatal versus postnatal.

respectively, which show that the trend was a decrease in overall negative emotion as well as a reduction in overall concerns for those with prenatal knowledge at the time of birth. Furthermore, positive emotions increased overall among parents with prenatal knowledge. This further demonstrates the better psychological preparedness that parents are equipped with when early prenatal counseling is offered.

ROLE OF MATERNAL-FETAL MEDICINE

MFM is the branch of obstetrics that focuses on the medical and surgical management of high-risk pregnancies. The Society for Maternal-Fetal Medicine recently released a special report to define the role of the MFM specialist in a health care setting. The Society clarifies that this subspecialist is an obstetrician-gynecologist who has completed 2 to 3 years of additional formal education and clinical training within an American Board of Obstetrics and Gynecology (ABOG)-approved or American Osteopathic Board of Obstetrics and Gynecology (AOBOG)-approved fellowship program and is eligible for or certified by ABOG or AOBOG as having a special competence in the diagnosis and treatment of women with complications of pregnancy. MFM subspecialists have the specific training and experience required to perform complex diagnostic and therapeutic procedures during pregnancy that can involve the mother and/or fetus. MFM specialists have advanced knowledge of the medical, surgical, obstetric, fetal, and genetic complications of pregnancy and their effects on both mother and fetus. Finally, they provide peer and patient education and perform research concerning the most recent approaches and treatments for obstetric problems, thus promoting risk-appropriate care for these complicated pregnancies.[14]

In the United States, MFM specialists are small in number and most are centered around major urban academic centers. This uneven distribution creates difficulties for women in certain geographic regions in obtaining consultation from an MFM specialist. A population survey conducted by the University of New Mexico looked at the MFM workforce in the United States. The investigators found that in 2010 there were 1355 MFM subspecialists currently working in the United States, with the highest number in the most populous states. Nearly all (98.2%) resided in metropolitan counties with level III perinatal centers.[15]

Despite their small numbers, they are able to provide a valuable service in the management of cleft lip and palate patients. They are able to provide targeted 3-D/4-D ultrasound imaging for making the diagnosis of a cleft lip. They are also able to perform complex procedures for advanced prenatal diagnosis, including chorionic villus sampling, amniocentesis for karyotyping, fluorescence in situ hybridization, and DNA analysis.

The ABOG has recently begun to adjust the education requirements for this subspecialty and, as its training becomes better defined, so will its role with the management of cleft lip and palate patients. At this time, it is the author's recommendation for cleft and craniofacial surgeons to work closely with this highly trained subspecialty whenever possible. Often MFM physicians are the first to interact with the parents of a cleft patient and often are the first to make the diagnosis. It is appropriate for a cleft team to seek out and invite an MFM specialist to participate as a dedicated member of a cleft team. It is prudent to have a combined prenatal counseling session involving both a surgeon and MFM specialist to introduce parents to the timeline of repairs for their upcoming child.

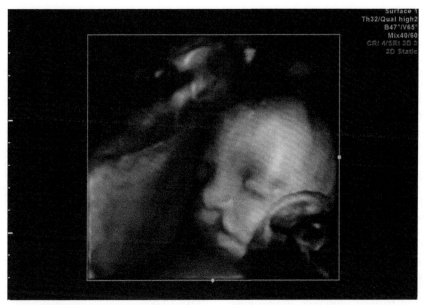

Fig. 3. Child with a cleft lip seen on 3-D ultrasound.

ULTRASONOGRAPHY

Since the late 1950s, prenatal ultrasound has been the workhorse of obstetric imaging. Its low-risk, high-yield nature has prompted clinicians to use this diagnostic modality for a host of intrauterine evaluation techniques. The role of 2-D transabdominal, transvaginal, or transperineal ultrasound examination in detecting congenital malformations during the second trimester has been well described.[16] More recently, 3-D/4-D sonography has been gaining wide acceptance in prenatal birthing centers. With addition of the sagittal plane, 3-D sonography is able to construct a computerized volumetric rendering of the fetus, in much the same way CT volumetric reconstructions are created. The difference between 3-D and 4-D is the time factor. The reconstruction of a 3-D image traditionally involves a time lag while the computer performs the reconstruction; however, when real-time image creation was introduced, the imaging was designated 4-D. **Fig. 3** shows an example of a child with a cleft lip seen on 3-D ultrasound, and Video 1 shows an example of real-time 4-D sonography.

A cleft deformity was first diagnosed by ultrasound and subsequently described in the literature by Christ and Meininger in 1981.[17] Since that time, the detection rates have rapidly improved in a linear fashion as computer technology has quickly advanced. Detection rates of the cleft anomaly that are reported in the literature should be circumspect to readers. Detection rates of up to 75% have been described by specialist MFM and radiology departments.[18,19] This is due to an inherent bias from referral patterns to these departments where the cohort of patients are often there for a second opinion from an initial diagnosis made at a birthing center.

Regardless, it is safe to assume that it is readily possible to make a prenatal diagnosis of cleft lip by 2-D high-definition ultrasound. The same cannot be said for diagnosing a cleft palate. This is an important consideration because although the prenatal counseling to the parents for an isolated cleft lip includes discussion of potentially a single surgical procedure to correct the soft tissue defect, variations in phenotype of the cleft palate result in an extremely diverse treatment regimen of multiple surgeries to correct feeding issues, speech difficulty, and iatrogenic maxillary growth restriction. Most ultrasonographers acknowledge an inability to visualize the posterior hard and soft palate using the traditional 2-D ultrasound scan. Recent advancement in 3-D and 4-D high-resolution ultrasound has helped improve, although not completely eradicate, the difficulty in visualizing the extent of the posterior palatal defect. It is important to recognize that there is a lack of uniform terminology in ultrasonography literature of what constitutes a cleft lip versus a cleft palate. Unfortunately, most reports on the success of prenatal 3-D ultrasound diagnosis of cleft lip and palate designate the cleft lip as involving soft tissue only, and when a cleft involves the bony alveolar ridge it is designated cleft palate. This is inherently misleading for the parents, for although the surgical correction of an isolated alveolar cleft is of minimal morbidity, the opposite is true for a cleft that extends through the posterior hard and soft palate. A more clear description appropriately used by some ultrasound investigators designates cleft lip as involving clefting of the lip, clefting of the premaxilla/alveolus, and clefting of the secondary hard palate. These same investigators report good rates of posterior bony cleft palate detection using 3-D/4-D ultrasound.[20] Most investigators, however, agree that a limitation of even 3-D/4-D ultrasound detection is the inability to visualize the extent of soft palate defect. The role of prenatal fetal MRI in further diagnosing the extent of palatal clefting is beyond the scope of this article; however, in the future its use may become more frequent in diagnosing the extent of the cleft anomaly.

Despite the clear advantage of using 3-D/4-D sonography as a screening tool, it has not gained widespread acceptance. Often cited is the lack of time needed to train clinicians during busy clinical schedules, lack of vendor support, cost of implementation, and maintenance of new hardware as well as clinicians' attitudes toward adapting and learning new technology.[21] The use of 3-D/4-D sonography in detection of cleft lip and palate is a technically difficult procedure and there is a steep learning curve for practitioners. Some reports in the literature describe this learning curve as a major hurdle to using 3-D/4-D sonography for routine diagnosis of cleft lip and palate patients. As previously discussed, the MFM physician is a uniquely positioned professional to receive advanced training in using and interpreting these modalities. Although educational requirements for MFM fellows continues to evolve, it is encouraging that a recent survey of MFM fellowship obstetric ultrasound experience showed that most responders describe being trained in 2-D as well as 3-D and 4-D ultrasound. The study also highlighted that most fellows begin their prenatal ultrasound training in the first year of fellowship and 80% to 100% of faculty perform prenatal ultrasound examinations routinely.[22] This finding further emphasizes the important role that MFM will continue to play in the comprehensive care of cleft patients.

SUMMARY

In conclusion, using a multidisciplinary team is of paramount importance when treating cleft lip and palate patients. Although it is not always feasible to include MFM physicians in the care of cleft patients due to regional availability, working with this highly skilled subspecialty whenever possible is highly encouraged. An MFM physician can offer valuable contributions to the initial diagnosis using advanced imaging and laboratory modalities as well as contribute to the prenatal counseling and treatment coordination for a patient's parents. Furthermore, obtaining a clearer prenatal image diagnosis of the extent of a cleft anomaly using 3-D/4-D ultrasonography is of benefit both in assisting surgeons in planning the necessary operations and improving parents' bonding with their children. As these advanced diagnostic modalities continue to evolve, so should oral and maxillofacial surgeons' knowledge of them so that they might use them in more thorough surgical planning.

SUPPLEMENTARY DATA

Supplementary data related to this article can be found online at http://dx.doi.org/10.1016/j.coms.2015.12.005.

REFERENCES

1. IPDTOC Working Group. Prevalence at birth of cleft lip with or without cleft palate. Data from the International Perinatal Database of Typical Oral Clefts (IPDTOC). Cleft Palate Craniofac J 2011;48:66–81.
2. Croen LA, Shaw GM, Wasserman CR, et al. Racial and ethnic variations in the prevalence of orofacial clefts in California, 1983-1992. Am J Med Genet 1998;79:42–7.
3. Marazita ML, Mooney MP. Current concepts in the embryology and genetics of cleft lip and cleft palate. Clin Plast Surg 2004;31:125–40.
4. American Cleft Palate-Craniofacial Association Parameters for evaluation and treatment of patients with cleft lip/palate or other craniofacial anomalies. Cleft Palate Craniofac J 1993;30(Supp 1):S1–16. Available at: http://www.acpa-cpf.org/uploads/site/Parameters_Rev_2009.pdf.
5. Strauss RP, ACPA Team Standards Committee. Cleft palate and craniofacial teams in the United States and Canada: a national survey of team organization and standards of care. Cleft Palate Craniofac J 1998;35(6):473–80.
6. Commission on Approval of Teams. Standards for approval of cleft palate and craniofacial teams. 2015. Available at: www.acpa-cpf.com. Accessed July 18, 2015.
7. Hunfeld JA, Tempels A, Passchier J, et al. Brief report, parental burden and grief one year after the birth of a child with a congenital anomaly. J Pediatr Psychol 1999;24:515–20.
8. Rey-Bellet C, Hohlfeld J. Prenatal diagnosis of facial clefts: evaluation of a specialized counseling. Swiss Med Wkly 2004;134:640–4.

9. Davalbhakta A, Hall PN. The impact of antenatal diagnosis on the effectiveness and timing of counselling for cleft lip and palate. Br J Plast Surg 2000;53:298–301.

10. Matthews MS, Cohen M, Viglione M, et al. Prenatal counselling for cleft lip and palate. Plast Reconstr Surg 1998;101:1–5.

11. da Silva Dalben G. Termination of pregnancy after prenatal diagnosis of cleft lip and palate - possible Influence on reports of prevalence. Oral Surg Oral Med Oral Pathol Oral Radiol Endod 2009;107:759–62.

12. Baker SR, Owens J, Stern M, et al. Coping strategies and social support in the family impact of cleft lip and palate and parents' adjustment and psychological distress. Cleft Palate Craniofac J 2009;46:229–36.

13. Berggren H, Hansson E, Uvemark A, et al. Prenatal compared with postnatal cleft diagnosis: what do the parents think? J Plast Surg Hand Surg 2012;46: 235–41.

14. Sciscione A, Berghella V, Blackwell S, et al. Society for maternal-fetal medicine (SMFM) special report: the maternal-fetal medicine subspecialists' role within a health care system. Am J Obstet Gynecol 2014;211(6):607–16.

15. Rayburn WF, Klagholz JC, Elwell EC, et al. Maternal-Fetal Medicine Workforce in the United States. Am J Perinatol 2012;29:741–6.

16. Chitty LS, Hunt GH, Moore J, et al. Effectiveness of routine ultrasonography in detecting fetal structural abnormalities in a low risk population. BMJ 1991; 303:1165–9.

17. Christ JE, Meininger MG. Ultrasound diagnosis of cleft lip and cleft palate before birth. Plast Reconstr Surg 1981;68:854–9.

18. Wayne C, Cook K, Sairam S, et al. Sensitivity and accuracy of routine antenatal ultrasound screening for isolated facial clefts. Br J Radiol 2002;75: 584–9.

19. Robinson JN, McElrath TF, Benson CB, et al. Prenatal ultrasonography and the diagnosis of fetal cleft lip. J Ultrasound Med 2001;20: 1165–70.

20. Rotten D, Levailiant JM. Two-and three-dimensional sonographic assessment of the fetal face. 2. Analysis of cleft lip, alveolus and palate. Ultrasound Obstet Gynecol 2004;24:402–11.

21. Ramos GA, Kfir M, Lee S, et al. Benefits of a systematic approach in the evaluation of fetal facial 3-dimensional volumes. J Ultrasound Med 2011;30: 473–9.

22. Blumenfeld YJ, Ness A, Platt LD. Maternal-fetal medicine fellowship obstetrical ultrasound experience: results from a fellowship survey. Prenat Diagn 2013;33:158–61.

Feeding Infants with Cleft and the Postoperative Cleft Management

David G. Gailey, DDS

KEYWORDS

- Cleft lip • Feeding • Cleft bottles • Feeding modifications • Wound care

KEY POINTS

- The development oral facial clefts can have a significant impact on the ability of the child to feed adequately.
- There are several feeding modifications available to help with normal feeding and aid in the normal development of oral-motor function.
- Postoperative wound care plays an essential part in cleft care; treatment providers should understand the wound healing pathway and ways it can be modified.

INTRODUCTION

Feeding in the cleft lip and palate setting is a major and continued challenge that parents, nurses and surgeon's encounter. Feeding is an important time in the neonate's life when the mother-child bond is developed. The infant is also developing the complex oral-motor skills required to accommodate future complex feeding and eventual speech development. Adequate feeding is vital for healthy infant development and growth. Feeding challenges are among the greatest concerns that parents and caretakers have during the initial stages of cleft diagnosis. Young and colleagues[1] demonstrated that 97% of parents thought that it was critical to discuss feeding challenges of cleft infants and 95% thought it was critical to have a demonstration of breast or bottle feeding. In the same study, only 55% of parents reported having feeding demonstrations during the cleft evaluation and 40% of parents were not informed of the potential feeding difficulties. Adequate nutrition in the presurgical and postsurgical phases of cleft care is invaluable. It is imperative that providers for cleft patients appropriately understand the feeding challenges encountered with cleft deformities, as well as adequately inform and instruct families about how to overcome those challenges.

Postoperative wound management continues to be a poorly researched realm in cleft care. There exists wide diversity in postsurgical wound management protocols and variability from differing surgeons and cleft centers. Research is challenging due to the lack of standardization of post-cleft repair along with the inherent genetic variations that affect scar development.

INFANT FEEDING AND SWALLOWING

Feeding and swallowing is an essential task that every neonate undertakes within the first hours of life. Neurologically intact infants are preprogramed with the innate knowledge of rooting along with the suck-swallow reflex. Rooting and sucking by the infant is stimulated by tactile stimulation to the mouth. Feeding is fundamental for adequate growth and development, along with oral-motor development. Feeding also serves as a time for bonding between mother and child and allows for the development of early communication skills as the infant responds to mother's cues. Infant-parent communication behaviors have a direct positive influence on the success of infant feeding performances.[2] Feeding action is also pivotal in the early development of oral-motor coordination and is the foundation of for future complex feeding

Inland Oral Surgery, 2204 East 29th Avenue, Suite #104, Spokane, WA 99203, USA
E-mail address: drgailey@inlandoralsurgery.com

Oral Maxillofacial Surg Clin N Am 28 (2016) 153–159
http://dx.doi.org/10.1016/j.coms.2015.12.003
1042-3699/16/$ – see front matter © 2016 Elsevier Inc. All rights reserved.

and speaking motions that will be developed. Cleft lip or palate malformations have the potential to disrupt a portion or all of the normal feeding process and, in turn, result in complex abnormalities for both the child and family.

Normal Anatomy and Physiology

There are several anatomic variations in the newborn anatomy that facilitate the sucking action. One of the main obvious differences is that most of the structures are smaller in size and closer to each other. As the infant grows there is an increase in connective tissue volume along with complex muscle and neural tissue development.[3] The infant tongue is relatively larger in size ratio to the oral cavity and fills most of the oral cavity. Infants have large buccal fat pads that aid to stabilize the lateral walls of the oral cavity. Because of the underdeveloped temporomandibular joint and lack of dentition, an infant's mouth opening is smaller and can be closed deeper than the adult mouth.[4] The soft palate in newborns tends to be longer and has a greater surface contact with the posterior portion of the tongue. Along with a closer approximation of the lateral pharyngeal walls, this makes the overall pharyngeal space smaller. In infants, the larynx is approximately one-third the size of the adult and is located high in the hypopharynx, causing the epiglottis to extend past the free margin of the soft palate. The epiglottis is more tubular and narrower than the adult structure and the tip often extends into the nasopharynx.[5] These anatomic variations facilitate sucking and improve the efficiency of the suck-swallow-breathing complex.

These anatomic differences directly aid in the physiologic process of feeding. A smooth, synchronized suck-swallow-breathing motion is key to adequate feeding and eventual growth and development. The swallow motion is separated into 2 phases: oral and the pharyngeal. The oral phase is initiated by rhythmic sucking. Anatomic structures create a pressure gradient as the tongue presses the nipple against the alveolar ridge while the lips create a seal around the nipple. As the nipple is compressed against the bony ridge, a positive pressure gradient is created, causing the release of fluid from the nipple. The infant initiates sucking by a rhythmic motion that involves the cupped tongue around the nipple moving in a backwards direction. The jaw drops, enlarging the oral cavity and creating a negative pressure gradient, causing more fluid to be expressed. Nipple compression against the alveolar ridge and generation of negative pressure are required for normal feeding.

The pharyngeal phase of swallowing begins as the fluid bolus is moved posterior from the oral cavity into the pharynx. As the pharyngeal phase begins, a variety of movements occur to allow the infant to continue nasal breathing during sucking, while avoiding laryngeal aspiration or nasal regurgitation of fluids. When the fluid bolus is moved posteriorly, the velum elevates to close the velopharyngeal valve. Due to the elongated epiglottis, the velum does not contact the posterior pharyngeal wall but instead closes around the epiglottis. This allows the infant to maintain nasal breathing during sucking. The tongue base moves posteriorly as negative pressure builds, moving the fluid bolus into the pharyngeal space around the epiglottis.[6] Once swallowing is initiated the epiglottis is retracted over the larynx by adduction of the laryngeal muscles, including the true and false vocal folds, as well as the arytenoid muscles.[7] The fluid bolus is advanced from the pharynx into the esophagus, initiating the esophageal phase. The esophagus has upper and lower esophageal sphincters that are closed during the oral and pharyngeal phases of swallowing. As the fluid bolus moves from the pharynx to the hypopharynx, the esophageal sphincters open and the fluid bolus is passed into the stomach. Once swallowing is complete, the velum drops, the epiglottis elevates, and the tongue moves back to a forward position. The upper and lower esophageal sphincters close and the process starts anew. Synchronization of the suck-swallow-breathing mechanism is critical to prevent aspiration or nasal regurgitation.

Feeding Challenges in Cleft Patients

As are the variations in cleft formation, feeding difficulties in patients with clefts are equally diverse. In the isolated cleft, not associated with syndrome, feeding problems result from the anatomic-structural deformity and usually only affect the oral phase of the suck-swallow-breathing mechanism. When the cleft is associated with a syndrome, the risk of poor feeding is 15 times more probable.[8] Feeding challenges include poor oral suction, inadequate volume intake, lengthy feeding time, nasal regurgitation, excessive air intake, coughing, or choking.[9] Feeding challenges are secondary to the inability to create nipple seal from the labial cleft, inadequate nipple compression due to nipple location on nasal mucosa versus the alveolar ridge, and inability to separate the oral and nasal cavities because of the hard palatal cleft. Patients with isolated labial clefts or small clefts of the soft palate can often create and maintain normal levels of suction and compression. When the cleft progresses and involves the complete lip, alveolar ridge, hard palate, or is bilateral, the ability to create adequate seal and suction is significantly decreased.[10] Most cleft infants have decreased sucking efficiency due to shorter sucks, faster sucking rate, a high suck–swallow ratio, and inability to generate adequate intraoral pressure. The decrease in sucking efficiency and poor feeding abilities lead to decreased oral intake, reduced weight gain, and inadequate growth.[11] Feeding difficulties also affect the interaction between the infant and caretaker and make feeding time stressful for both.

Feeding difficulties have a detrimental effect on growth and development in the cleft infant. Infants require 2 to 3 ounces of breast milk or formula per pound of body weight per day to supply adequate nutrition requirements to ensure normal development.[12] In most infants this correlates to 20 to 30 ounces of fluid per day, which can be challenging for a cleft infant and caregiver who is having feeding difficulties. Evaluating the volume of breast milk or formula a cleft infant is receiving is difficult due to nasal regurgitation or spit up from excessive air intake. Cleft infants usually take longer to achieve this volumetric goal. Babies are expected to gain, on average, 0.17 kg per week from 0 to 12 weeks of age.[13] This increase in effort and energy adds an additional caloric need and often negates the added fluid intake. The increased effort leaves the cleft infant with a caloric deficit, which results in delayed growth. Most feedings should take 20 to 30 minutes.[4] Feedings taking 45 minutes or longer require additional observation with a feeding specialist as well as a pediatrician to ensure adequate weight gain.

Feeding Modifications

The goals of feeding modifications are to ensure the cleft infant has adequate nutritional supply to allow for normal development. The modified feeding technique should be as close to normal as possible to allow for normal development of oral-motor functions. Because cleft malformations have wide variations, feeding interventions should be equally unique. A wide variety of cleft feeding modifications are available, including nipple shields, supplemental nursing systems, modified nipples, and oral obturators. Individual assessment with a feeding specialist during the initial feeding with the mother will dictate which technique is best for the infant.

Most pediatricians and health care providers recommend breastfeeding. Breast milk contains the mother's antibodies, which aid in protecting against illness, helps in avoiding early food allergies, and has been suggested to protect from otitis media.[14] Breastfeeding also proves beneficial in the child–mother bond formation. The ability to breastfeed varies depending on the size and location of the cleft as well as the mother's flow of milk. Cleft patients with isolated incomplete labial clefts can often be successful with breastfeeding. Nipple shields can be used if the infant demonstrates difficulties with latching. Nipple shields are made of thin, pliable silicone and allow the infant to latch more easily to the breast (**Fig. 1**). They also assist in forming a seal to increase suction. Breastfeeding becomes much more challenging with palatal clefts due to the inability to create adequate suction. Patients need to be closely monitored and counseled if weight gain is not demonstrated.

When feeding difficulties are immediately identified, feedings using specialty bottles are ideal to ensure adequate nutritional intake. Specialty bottles improve feeding efficiency as well as aid in the oral-motor development. Most modifications are made through the nipple. Increasing pliability, changing the nipple shape and size, and modifications to the nipple hole diameter facilitate feeding. Each of the nipple characteristics is determined by the infant's ability to complete each phase of the suck-swallow-breathing mechanism. In general, a more pliable nipple correlates to an increased rate of fluid flow. Nipple shapes vary from traditional to flat, and broad to thin. The nipple shape is important in supporting the oral-motor patterns of sucking. Correct nipple size is important to maintain adequate contact with the tongue during sucking. The size and type of nipple hole affect the flow rate. Crosscut holes allow much more fluid flow from the nipple and only allow flow during compression. Often, newborn infants are not able to tolerate the increased flow released from crosscut nipples. This results in increased coughing and nasal reflux. Traditional nipple holes allow for milk to

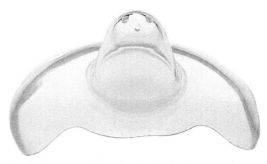

Fig. 1. Nipple shield used to facilitate latching to breast.

drip steadily from the nipple tip. In addition to modified nipple tips, flexible bottles can be used to aid in cleft feeding. Flexible bottles allow the feeder to assist the infant in expressing milk into the mouth, decreasing effort and conserving energy. Synchronization between the caretaker and baby are critical to the success of this type of feeding.

Bottles commonly used for feeding infants with cleft deformities include the Cleft Palate Nurser, Mead Johnson LLC, Glenview, IL; Medela Special-Needs Feeder, formerly the Haberman bottle (Medela, Inc Breastfeeding U.S., McHenry, IL, USA); Pigeon Bottle (Philips, Amsterdam, The Netherlands); and vented bottles such as the Dr Brown Bottle (Dr Brown's, St Louis, MO, USA). Each feeding system has advantages along with disadvantages.

The Cleft Palate Nurser is considered an assisted-delivery bottle. The bottle is made of a soft plastic that is easily compressible. The caregiver is able to squeeze the bottle and assist fluid flow to the infant. The disadvantage is that it requires coordination between the infant and feeder to prevent forced swallowing during rest and coughing.

The Medela SpecialNeeds Feeder is an assisted-delivery bottle (**Fig. 2**). It is designed for infants who have minimal sucking ability. The bottle is composed of 5 parts that include a valve, disk, nipple, collar, and bottle. The milk is drawn in from the bottle to the nipple. The valve keeps the milk in the nipple. When the infant compresses the nipple tip, milk freely flows. The nipple has 3 markings on the side that correspond to increased milk flow rate. The nipple can also be compressed to allow the feeder to express increased volumes. This bottle is a common feeding system in cleft care due to the versatility to compensate for the wide range in cleft defects and the relative ease of use.

Pigeon Bottles (**Fig. 3**) are composed of 4 parts, including a plastic 1-way valve, nonlatex nipple with a Y-cut hole and vent, collar, and a bottle. The Pigeon nipple is soft on 1 side and firm on the other. The firm side is placed on the roof of the mouth and the soft side against the infants tongue. The small notch on the nipple indicates the location of the air vent and should be pointing up. The 1-way valve is placed with the flat side toward the nipple and functions to keep milk in the nipple. Due to the crosscut nipple hole, it has a faster flow rate than the SpecialNeeds Feeder and can be difficult for newborns.[15]

Vented bottles, such as the Dr Brown bottle (**Fig. 4**), are made with an internal vent that is believed to decrease negative pressures and reduce air bubbles that occur during feeding. Elimination of negative pressure is believed decrease the amount of air the infant swallows, which in turn reduces colic, spit-up, burping, and gas. There are few studies that actually confirm this effect.

It is imperative that the caregiver work closely with a lactation and feeding specialist to ensure the infant is obtaining adequate nutritional intake

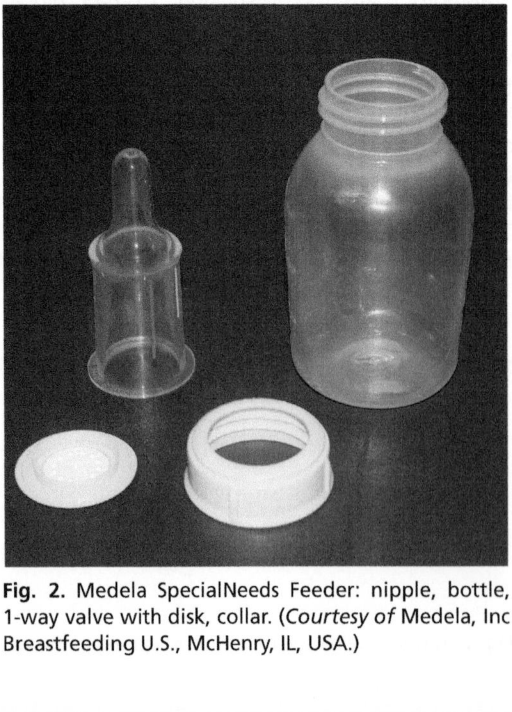

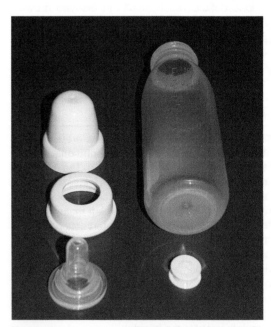

Fig. 2. Medela SpecialNeeds Feeder: nipple, bottle, 1-way valve with disk, collar. (*Courtesy of* Medela, Inc Breastfeeding U.S., McHenry, IL, USA.)

Fig. 3. Pigeon system: collar, bottle, pigeon nipple, plastic 1-way valve. (*Courtesy of* Philips, Amsterdam, The Netherlands.)

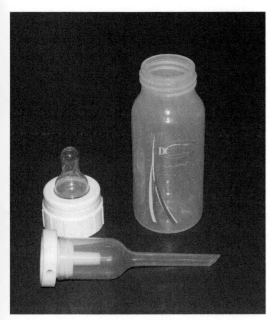

Fig. 4. Dr Brown system: nipple with collar, bottle, internal vent. (*Courtesy of* Dr Brown's, St Louis, MO, USA.)

to allow for normal growth. Another, often overlooked, challenge that families encounter is the cost associated with specialty feeding systems. Most of these feeding devices range in price from $20 to $30 per bottle. The associated cost can add additional stress to the families and caregivers of cleft children. Most cleft teams have established grants to help families in need that could otherwise be unable to obtain these vital feeding methods.

Postoperative Feeding

For many parents the feeding challenges start anew once the surgical correction of the cleft deformity is complete. Feeding protocols in the postoperative period continue to be a controversial subject among cleft teams. Many cleft centers use postsurgical feeding protocols that lack evidence of effectiveness. Many centers and surgeons recommend 3 to 5 days of bottle holiday during the postoperative phase and use syringe feeds. Studies demonstrate that the mechanical effects of feeding have little effect on wound complications or incision breakdown.[16–20] Nutritional intake plays a much larger role in wound complications than the mechanical motions involved with feeding. Returning to normal presurgical feeding regimens aids in continued nutritional intake for the infant as well as decreased feeding confusion for both the caretaker and the child.

POSTOPERATIVE WOUND CARE

Variation in postoperative wound management parallels the variation in surgical treatment options in cleft surgery. The commonality that all surgical interventions have is that they will inevitably leave evidence of repair in the form of a scar. Postoperative wound management plays a vital component in cleft management. Wound healing and scarring start with the initial stroke of the scalpel. The complex mechanism that allows wound regeneration includes inflammation, proliferation, and tissue remodeling. During the inflammatory phase, neutrophils and macrophages accumulate at the wound site to prevent infection.[21] Fibroblasts are recruited during the proliferative phase and begin synthesizing extracellular matrix molecules. These matrix molecules are haphazardly arranged to restore skin structure and function. Remodeling is the final phase of wound development. During this process, the extracellular matrix molecules are resorbed and new molecules deposited in a more formal and crosslinked arrangement. The proliferative phase accounts for most time required in scar tissue maturation.[22]

Scar development is an inevitable result of surgical treatment. The goal of postoperative wound management is to modify scar development and avoid unaesthetic scarring. This is especially important in the realm of cleft repair due to the location of the anticipated scar. Scar development is variable and can be influenced by anatomic location, size, severity, additional injury, and genetic predisposition.[23]

Scars are typically classified into 4 categories: fine line, hypertrophic, intermediate raised dermal, and keloids. The latter 3 share the commonality of demonstrating an overexpression of extracellular matrix molecules during the both the proliferative and remodeling phases. Keloids are distinct from normal scarring by the progression of the scar tissue beyond the original scar borders. Keloids also do not tend to regress over time.[24]

This article is not meant to be an all-inclusive review of scar treatment but, instead, an overview of the more common treatment options in the immediate postsurgical setting. Several topical medications have been used to aid favorable scar formation. Medications include vitamin E, onion extract, calcium channel blockers, and immune response modulators. Each treatment is aimed to modify a portion of the wound healing process to enable the scar to both look and feel like adjacent tissue. There are few randomized control studies that measure the effectiveness of each of these treatment options.

Vitamin E is a commonly used, topically applied, medication for improved scar formation. It has been used for decades as a moisturizer and anti-oxidant to decrease the inflammatory effect in the scarring process as well as to help prevent ultraviolet damage. Studies have failed to substantiate these effects. Regardless of lack of clinical evidence, it remains the most commonly prescribed postoperative topical medication for wound healing.[25]

Onion extract and immune response modifiers are believed to improve scar formation by reducing the expression of extracellular matrix molecules during the proliferation phase of wound healing. A decrease in the total number of extracellular matrix molecules results in a decrease in scar stiffness and a scarring that feels more similar to the adjacent tissue.[23] Calcium channel blockers have also been used to decrease the proliferation of extracellular matrix molecules. Calcium channel blockers affect the remodeling phase of wound healing by stimulating procollagen synthesis. This, in turn, decreases collagen deposits and decreases the total stiffness of the scar tissue. Most studies demonstrating these effects are in vitro or case reports. Few randomized in vivo studies are available to collaborate the clinical effects of these commonly used medications.[23]

The author's preference for postoperative wound management includes modification of both the inflammatory and proliferative phases of wound healing. Initial wound development is allowed for 2 weeks after surgical repair of facial cleft. The caregiver is then instructed to use gentle massage to apply onion extract to the surgical site twice a day, once in the morning and once at night. The massage has the theoretic benefits of allowing deeper penetration of the medication into the forming scar tissue along with a mechanical softening of the newly deposited extracellular matrix molecules. After application of onion extract, a small bead of silicone gel is applied to the scar line. This hydrates the scar, which, in turn, aids in improved scar condition and color. One of more challenging decisions for the surgeon is to do nothing when presented with an unfavorable aesthetic scar. The surgeon must resist the urge to perform repeated revision surgeries on unaesthetic scars. Repeated surgery restarts the wound healing process and removes the most important variable in scar development: time.

SUMMARY

Cleft lip and palate malformations have diverse clinical presentations. Most clefts affect the ability to adequately feed, which can be detrimental to growth and development. Feeding difficulties associated with cleft formation need to be discussed with the parents or caregivers early and addressed often to maintain adequate infant health. Many cleft feeding modifications are available to cleft families. Choosing the appropriate feeding technique must be individualized to allow normal function of the suck-swallow-breathing mechanism, as well as the development of oral-motor function. Feeding in the postsurgical setting should be returned to normal as soon as possible to maintain adequate nutritional intake and allow for good wound healing.

Postoperative wound care is an essential component to cleft repair. Cleft surgeons should understand the complex mechanism of wound healing along with options of how to augment the process to achieve aesthetic scar healing.

REFERENCES

1. Young JL, O'Riordan M, Goldstein JA, et al. What information do parents of newborns with cleft lip, palate, or both want to know? Cleft Palate Craniofac J 2001;38(1):55–8.
2. Meyer EC, Coll CT, Lester BM, et al. Family-based interventions improve maternal psychological well-being and feeding interactions of preterm infants. Pediatrics 1994;93(2):241–6.
3. Bosma JF. Postnatal ontogeny of performances of the pharynx, larynx, and mouth. Am Rev Respir Dis 1985;131:S10–5.
4. Kummer AW. Cleft palate and craniofacial anomalies, effects on speech and resonance. 2nd edition. Clifton Park (NY): Delmar Cengage Learning; 2008.
5. Myer CM, Cotton RT, Shott SR. The pediatric airway: an interdisciplinary approach. Philadelphia: J.B. Lippincott; 1995.
6. Newman LA, Cleveland RH, Blickman JG, et al. Videofluoroscopic analysis of the infant swallow. Invest Radiol 1991;26(10):870–3.
7. Koeing JS, Davies AM, Thach BT. Coordination of breathing, sucking and swallowing during bottle feedings in human infants. J Appl Physiol (1985) 1990;69:1623–9.
8. Reid J, Kilpatrick N, Reilly S. A prospective, longitudinal study of the feeding skills in a cohort of babies with cleft conditions. Cleft Palate Craniofac J 2006; 43(6):702–9.
9. Masarei AG, Sell D, Habel A, et al. The nature of feeding in infants with unrepaired cleft lip and/or palate compared with healthy noncleft infants. Cleft Palate Craniofac J 2007;44(3):321–8.
10. Reid J, Reilly S, Kilpatrick N. Sucking performance of babies with cleft conditions. Cleft Palate Craniofac J 2007;33(3):312–20.

11. Carlisle D. Feeding babies with cleft lip and palate. Nurs Times 1998;94(4):59–60.

12. The Cleft Palate Foundation. Feeding an infant with a cleft. Chapel Hill (NC): Author; 1998.

13. Ize-Iyamu IN, Saheeb BD. Feeding intervention in cleft lip and palate babies; a practical approach to feeding efficiency and weight gain. Int J Oral Maxillofac Surg 2011;40:916–9.

14. Aniansson G, Svensson H, Becker M, et al. Otitis media and feeding with breast milk of children with cleft palate. Scand J Plast Reconstr Surg 2002;36:9–15.

15. Available at: http://www.seattlechildrens.org/medical-conditions/chromosomal-genetic-conditions/cleft-lip-palate-feeding/. Accessed August, 2015.

16. Cohen M, Marschall MA, Schafer ME. Immediate unrestricted feeding of infants following cleft lip and palate repair. J Craniofac Surg 1992;3(1):30–2.

17. Kim EK, Lee TJ, Chae SW. Effect of unrestricted bottle-feeding on early postoperative course cleft palate repair. J Craniofac Surg 2009;20(Suppl 2):1886–8.

18. Trettene Ados S, Mondini CC, Marques IL, et al. Feeding children in the immediate perioperative period after palatoplasty; a comparison between techniques using a cup and spoon. Rev Esc Enferm USP 2013;47(6):1298–304. Available at: www.ee.usp.br/reeusp/.

19. Hughes J, Lindup M, Wright S, et al. Does nasogastric feeding reduce distress after cleft palate repair in infants? Nurs Child Young People 2013;25(9):26–30.

20. Skinner J, Arvedson JC, Jones G, et al. Post-operative feeding strategies for infants with cleft lip. Int J Pediatr Otorhinolaryngol 1997;42(2):169–78.

21. Eming SA, Krieg T, Davidson JM. Inflammation in wound repair; molecular and cellular mechanisms. J Invest Dermatol 2007;127(3):514–25.

22. Clark RA. Fibrin and wound healing. Ann N Y Acad Sci 2001;936:355–67.

23. Byat A, McGrouther DA, Ferguson MW. Skin scarring. BMJ 2003;326(7380):88–92.

24. Sidgwick GP, McGeorge D, Bayat AA. Comprehensive evidence-based review on the role of topicals and dressing in the management of skin scarring. Arch Dermatol Res 2015;307:461–77.

25. Curran JN, Crealey M, Sadadcharam G, et al. Vitamin E: patterns of understanding, use, and prescription by health professionals and students at a university teaching hospital. Plast Reconstr Surg 2006;118(1):248–52.

Presurgical Orthopedics Appliance
The Latham Technique

Carlos Cruz, DDS

KEYWORDS

• Orthopedics • Appliance • Surgery • Latham technique

KEY POINTS

- The Latham technique is a procedure used to treat facial orthopedic abnormalities in unilateral and bilateral cleft lip and palate patients.
- The Latham appliance applies controlled direction that forces the repositioning of the displaced basal segments and realigns soft tissue margins prior to corrective surgery.
- The Latham pinning technique obtains anchorage from the base of the maxilla to affect orthopedic repositioning of the cleft maxillary segments or premaxilla.
- The Latham appliances have proven to be successful in expanding and aligning the maxillary segments, retruding a protruded premaxilla, aligning bilateral alveolar ridges, creating less tension on surgical closure and statistically reduction of fistulas.
- The Latham device is a valuable pre-operative tool for a surgeon when treating cleft defects. In selective cases (wide cleft and severe protruded pre-maxilla) surgery alone is more aggressive and a less controlled treatment.

BACKGROUND

Presurgical orthopedics (PSO) for neonates originated in the sixteenth century; Franco was the first to describe the use of a headcap to retract a protruded premaxilla.[1,2] Various other extraoral concepts were documented in the decades to follow; Hoffmann in 1686, Louis in 1768, Chaussier in 1776, Desault in 1790, Hullinhen in 1844, Thiesch in 1875, and Von Esmarch and Kowalzig in 1892.[1,2]

In 1927, Brophy developed an intraoral approach; he described passing wires through the ends of the cleft alveolus, and tightening the wires to reduce the cleft.[1,2] Three decades later, McNeil and Burston were first to describe a concept using a series of modified acrylic appliances; each successive appliance was fabricated with the cleft gap slightly closer.[1,3] McNeil's technique was successful at closing the alveolar gap and the hard palate cleft; this novel approach to controlled alveolar movement is now seen as the beginning of modern PSO.[1–6] Since then, PSO appliances have evolved to the pin-retained expandable stainless steel bar described by Hagerty in 1957,[3,7] Georgiade and Mladick in 1968, Georgiade in 1970 and 1971, Georgiade and Latham in 1975, and Latham in 1980.[1,3,8]

Since the 1980s, many cleft centers have adopted the Latham technique as the initial intervention used to treat cleft lip and palate defects. In 2005, Weinfeld and colleagues[9] reported on the international tenets of cleft treatment. He stated that most participating cleft centers used presurgical appliances; of this group, 24.3% used the Latham appliance, a 5% increase from the previous survey in 2000.[9] Most recently, Tan and colleagues (2012)[10] reported that 71% of 241 surgeons surveyed used PSO; although no exact value was given, the Latham appliance was the second most commonly used.

THE TECHNIQUE

The first step in the rehabilitation of a newborn with a cleft defect is taking a maxillary impression (**Fig. 1**); at this point the infant is usually 2 weeks

Oral & Craniofacial Center, PLLC, 2405 Cornerstone Boulevard, Edinburg, TX 78539, USA
E-mail address: ccruz@drcruzoms.com

Oral Maxillofacial Surg Clin N Am 28 (2016) 161–168
http://dx.doi.org/10.1016/j.coms.2016.01.004
1042-3699/16/$ – see front matter © 2016 Elsevier Inc. All rights reserved.

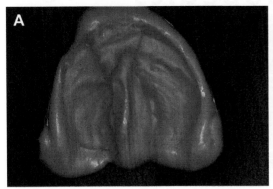 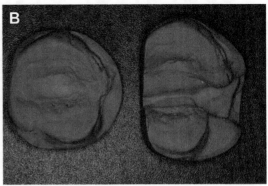

Fig. 1. (*A*) Intraoral impression of a unilateral cleft lip and palate in an infant, taken with polyvinylsiloxane material to capture the alveolar and palatal anatomy. (*B*) The impressions are used to create a precise stone cast model.

old or older.[11] Depending on the dynamics of the cleft team, this part of the treatment can be performed by the surgeon, pediatric dentist, or orthodontist. A master cast is produced and will be used in the fabrication of the pinned presurgical orthopedic (POC) device at either the doctor's or a specialty dental laboratory.

Although the delivery of POC appliance is a quick procedure, it is done under general anesthesia and as early as 5 weeks of age.[11] The 2 maxillary bases are affixed by 2 channel-locking pins each; these pass through the acrylic material into the palate for intraosseous retention (**Fig. 2**).[6] After insertion of the POC device, the infant is typically monitored overnight and discharged the following morning. Now, the procedure is able to be performed as an outpatient surgery.

UNILATERAL CLEFT LIP AND PALATE

In unilateral cleft lip and palate (UCLP) treatment, once the appliance is placed and the patient is at home, the drive screw is activated one-half turn (0.25-mm displacement) twice a day by the parents (**Fig. 3**). The alignment of the alveolar segments depends on the size of the cleft, rate of activation, and amount of correction attempted (up to 14 mm).[6] Typically it takes around 3 to 6 weeks for the cleft side of the appliance to move forward with respect to the opposite side.[3] Throughout the alignment period, the surgeon evaluates the patient weekly until no further turning of the screw is possible. If the remaining gap between the segments exceeds 2 to 3 mm, an elastomeric chain is used across the front of the

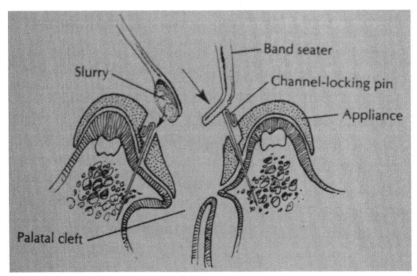

Fig. 2. Cross section showing intraosseous fixation of the base appliance to the palatal shelves. A band seater and mallet are used to drive the 0.028 stainless steel channel-locking pins into the friction-fitting box channel of the acrylic base appliance. Carried by a spatula, a slurry of cold-cured acrylic is luted over each pinhead. (*From* Spolyar JL, Jackson IT, Sullivan W, et al. The Latham technique: contemporary presurgical orthopedics for the complete oral cleft technique and preliminary evaluation — a bone marker study. Semin Plast Surg 1992;6(1):182; with permission.)

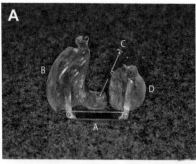
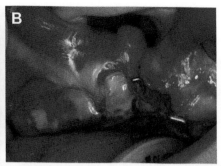

Fig. 3. (*A*) Dento-maxillary advancement appliance (DMA). The hinge allows the greater and lesser maxillary alveolar segments to rotate and translate to join them together. Turning the screw will activate the maxillary alveolar segments. The greater segment (B) will retreat with inward rotation and the lesser segment (D) will auto-rotate and advance to join the segments together. (*B*) Prior to reconstructive surgery and removal of the appliance. The maxillary alveolar segments are aligned and approximated together. (*From* Spolyar JL, Jackson IT, Sullivan W, et al. The Latham technique: contemporary presurgical orthopedics for the complete oral cleft technique and preliminary evaluation — a bone marker study. Semin Plast Surg 1992;6(1):179–210.)

appliance (**Fig. 4**). A resting period of 2 to 3 weeks is recommended with the device still inserted after ideal movement is achieved; this dissipates residual load (strain) that builds up after applying the active force (stress).[6] Around the age of 3 months, the removal of the POC device is done under general anesthesia, and the surgeon can perform reconstructive surgery (**Fig. 5**).

BILATERAL CLEFT LIP AND PALATE

In bilateral cleft lip and palate (BCLP) correction, the maxillary acrylic bases are fixed to the palate in the same surgical manner as in UCLP but also with an additional premaxillary component. The acrylic bases expand the cleft segments and serve as anchors for the premaxillary retraction force. The surgeon places a staple through the septal premaxilla, and attaches it with the chains that proceed posteriorly under and around the roller below the expansion drive box (**Fig. 6 and 7**).[3] If a maxillary segment is needed, one-quarter turn twice a day by the parents is done or several one-quarter turns by the surgeon during the weekly checkups. The chains are shortened and checked by the surgeon weekly; they should only generate about 57 g (2 oz) of force. If the chains have excessive or uneven tension, the septal staple may be pulled without orthopedic effects and may fail. The desired pre-maxillary alignment is usually achieved in 4 to 6 weeks.[3] As with UCLP, a waiting period of 2 to 3 weeks is recommended. In addition, a deviated septum can be corrected by adding a wire islet to the palatal margin adjacent and opposite to the deviated vomer (**Fig. 8**). Around the age of 3 months, the removal of the POC device is done under general anesthesia, and the surgeon can perform reconstructive surgery (**Figs 8 and 9**).

BENEFITS

In 1987 Dr Ralph Millard, a prominent plastic surgeon and strong advocate for the Latham

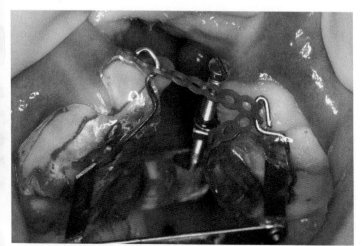

Fig. 4. Pinned dento-maxillary device (DMA) fully activated without complete closure of a wide defect. An elastic chain was used across the defect to rotate the segments medially to achieve a near-contact relationship. Chain strain should not exceed 57 to 85 g (2–3 oz).

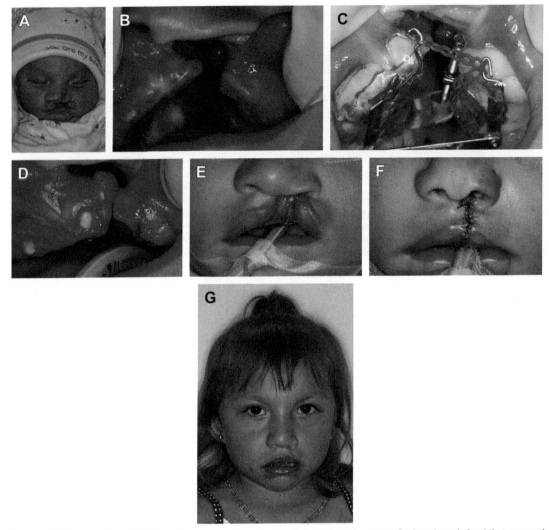

Fig. 5. (*A*) Facial view of left wide complete cleft lip. (*B*) Intraoral view of alveolar cleft. (*C*) Intraoral view of orthopedic appliance. (*D*) Approximation to an ideal arch alignment and removal of appliance before surgery. (*E*) Prior to lip and nose repair. (*F*) Cheilorhinoplasty. (*G*) Frontal view at follow-up after 1 year.

technique, described the surgical problems attending oral clefts without PSO.[3,12]

1. The lip closure alone does not reposition the premaxillary in BCLP or pull the cleft maxillary segment forward in UCLP well enough for closure of the cleft.
2. Persistent anterior fistulas present difficulty in surgical closure and in maintaining the patients' general well-being.
3. A protruded premaxilla at the base of the columella makes columellar lengthening and nasal tip correction impossible until the patient reaches adolescence.
4. Persistent fistulas and residual clefts in the alveolus require the difficult surgery of bone

grafting when the patient is between 6 and 8 years of age.
5. Satisfactory results have been achieved without PSO but the patient suffers through many years of misery.

Furthermore, Millard and colleagues[12] also listed the benefits of PSO[6]:

1. A better platform is produced for the lip and nose as well as for the alveolus.
2. Primary surgical closures can be performed without tension.
3. A more precise method controls the cleft components rather than the dependence on the

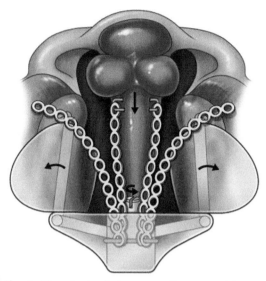

Fig. 6. The elastic chain premaxillary repositioning (ECPR) appliance is a means to both expand the maxillary base and anchor the premaxillary retraction chain force. The screw at the drive box is activated through the front of the mouth. Bilateral chains attached to the premaxilla pass under and around the drive box roller and then proceed forward and laterally to hook onto buttons at the head of each segment. (*From* Mulliken JB. Repair of bilateral cleft lip. In: Neligan P, editor. Plastic surgery. 3rd edition. Philadelphia (PA): Elsevier; 2013. p. 550–68; with permission.)

simple closure of the lip over the deformity to mold the distorted parts.

4. Dissection of mucoperiosteum at the edge of the cleft facilitates a 2-layer closure without tension.
5. Alveolar integrity is established to facilitate dental development.
6. Closure of the hard and soft palate is facilitated.
7. An intact primary palate is achieved at an early age.

8. A normal maxillary arch without fistulas is achieved with early secondary palate closure. Early fork-flap columellar surgery is possible in BCLP and can produce a good nose and lip.
9. Gingivoperiosteoplasty can be done with or without primary bone grafting.

Ever since Dr Ralph Millard's endorsement of the Latham technique in 1985, the PSO approach has been at the center of much debate; since then, the published research has focused on the long-term effects of the device. Out of the available trials, few are randomized controlled clinical trials (RCCT)[2,13]; furthermore, the general lack of objectivity and proper study design in these trials has let to questionable conclusions.[2,5,13]

In 1999, Millard and colleages[14] published the results of their study on PSO followed by periosteoplasty and lip adhesion (POPLA). Their article compared the results obtained using POPLA (group I) with those using the previous method (lip adhesion alone; group II) for cases of unilateral and bilateral clefts.[14] They acknowledged that there was a greater frequency of anterior crossbite in the POPLA group; however, the POPLA approach achieved the main goal of moving the palate into a normal position and stabilizing the arch with a bony bridge that attracts teeth. It avoids the difficult anterior fistulae and presents a more symmetric platform on which the lip can be united and the nose can be corrected early.[14] In 2007, Latham[15] reported a modification of the surgical protocol of BCLP that reduced the crossbite incidence from 83% to 33%.

In 2005, Berkowitz[16] published an article on the Latham-Millard technique (POPLA) and its adverse effects on facial growth; he used data from cleft patients treated from 1960 to 1980. Berkowitz[16] compared dental casts of patients treated with

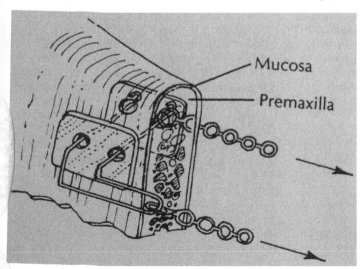

Mucosa

Premaxilla

Fig. 7. The retraction staple and polyethylene washers are placed through the pre-maxillary septal bone, which is prepared for staple insertion by drilling transverse holes aligned anteroposteriorly 3mm apart. Pre-maxillary retraction is initiated through a pulling action from a staple passed through the septal premaxilla. (*From* Mulliken JB. Repair of bilateral cleft lip. In: Neligan P, editor. Plastic surgery. 3rd edition. Philadelphia (PA): Elsevier; 2013. p. 550–68; with permission.)

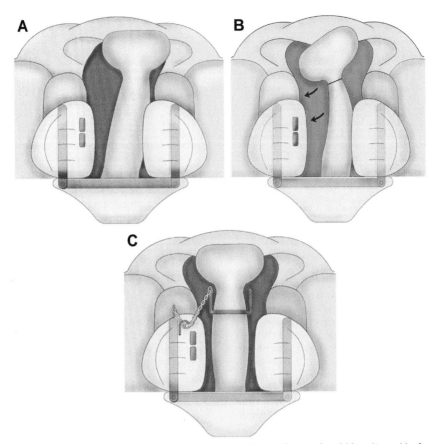

Fig. 8. (*A*) Deviated nasal septum. If the vomer is displaced to the midline it should be aligned before repositioning. This septal straightening method was originated by Dr. John Spolyar, Sterling Heights, Michigan USA. (*B*) Deviated nasal septum will bend at the premaxilla vomerine suture as force is applied to the pre-maxilla. (*C*) The modification of the ECPR is created by adding an islet at the opposite palatal base to the deviated vomer. A through and through pin is passed posterior to premaxilla and vomerian suture and the elastic chain through the loop at the islet at the palatal base to the anterior hook. Tension to the elastic will pull septum to the midline. At this moment the ECPR can be activated for better control. (*Courtesy of* John L. Spolyar, DDS, MS; Dr. Ralph Latham, London, Ontario, Canada.)

POPLA with those that did not receive the PSO approach. Berkowitz[16] reported that, in complete bilateral and UCLP, the frequency of the anterior crossbite and (except for ages 3 and 12 years) the buccal crossbite is significantly higher with the Latham-Millard PSO, gingivoperiosteoplasty, and lip adhesion protocol compared with the conservative, non-PSO without gingivoperiosteoplasty treatment.[16]

Uzel and Alparslan[13] (2011) pointed out that, in Millard and colleages'[14] and Berkowitz's[16] studies, the different surgical protocols make it difficult to determine whether the long-term results (crossbites) are caused by the PSO or the surgical techniques. What is not challenged in the conclusion is that the Latham device helps "avoid the difficult anterior fistulae and presents a more symmetrical platform upon which the lip can be united and the nose can be corrected early."[14]

Uzel and Alparslan[13] (2011) published the first systematic review on the long-term effects of PSO on cleft lip and palate; they mentioned only 7 RCCT that tested the Latham device. Out of the 7 Latham RCCT, only the trial by Chan and colleagues[21] (2003) was considered to have an adequate level of evidence. The remaining trials either for or against the Latham device, such as Roberts-Harry (1996), Henkel and Gundlach (1998), Millard (1999), Berkowitz (2004), Grisius (2006), and Latham (2007), are all excluded because of the different surgical or comparison protocols.[13]

The second systematic review, by Rani and colleagues[2] (2015), evaluates current literature on pre-surgical orthopedic (PSO) appliances; it addresses the Millard-Latham techniques among others. Rani and colleagues[2] concluded that the technique does not present either positive or negative long-term effects on maxillary growth.

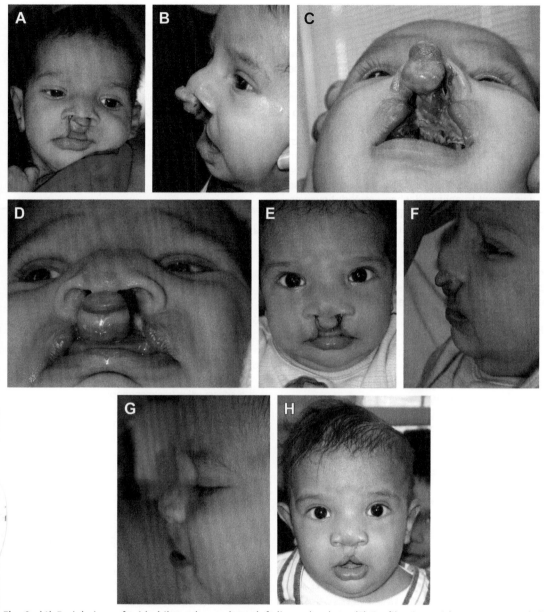

Fig. 9. (*A*) Facial view of wide bilateral complete cleft lip and palate. (*B*) Profile view with severe protruded premaxilla. (*C*) Occlusal view with intraoral orthopedic appliance. (*D–F*) Occlusal views of the child with intraoral orthopedic appliance; note that the premaxilla has moved mesioposteriorly in intraoral alignment. The columella is well visualized with the nasal complex structure. (*G, H*) Postoperative views, 3 months after cheilorhinoplasty.

Once more, the immediate presurgical advantages are not challenged to date.

Overall, Uzel and Alparslan[13] (2011) and Rani and colleagues[2] (2015) state that:

1 Well-structured standardized, longitudinal studies treating similar cleft defects and using the same management protocols are needed in order to achieve more conclusive data.[2,13]

2 Regarding the previous claims that PSO devices can cause unfavorable changes in the arch form and maxillary growth, and that they are complex, expensive, ineffective, and unnecessary: "None of these claims are evidence based."[2,13]

WHAT IS KNOWN

First introduced in 1980, the Latham appliance is classified as an active PSO device used for cleft defects. Its long-term effects are still debated; this is furthered by the lack of relevant clinical evidence on its use. The Latham device was introduced as a presurgical device to help surgeons achieve a more predictable surgical outcome; hence, it should be evaluated for its presurgical benefits. The device has been proved to be successful in expanding and aligning the maxillary segments; retruding protruded premaxillae; aligning bilateral alveolar ridges; and placing less tension on surgical closures; and, statistically, it reduces the rate of fistulation from between 20% and 50% down to 8%.[6,17–20] The Latham device has provided the presurgical value it was meant to achieved when created; however, it has not been shown to have either a positive or negative long-term effect on maxillary development or occlusion.[21] Overall, the Latham device is a valuable preoperative tool for surgeons treating cleft defects. In selective cases (wide clefts and severe protruded premaxilla) surgery alone is a more aggressive and less controlled treatment.

REFERENCES

1. Grabb WC, Smith JW, Aston SJ, et al. Presurgical orthopedics for cleft lip and palate. In: Grabb and Smith's plastic surgery. 5th edition. Philadelphia: Lippincott-Raven; 1997. p. 237–44.

2. Rani ST, Rajendra RE, Manjula M, et al. Diversities in presurgical orthopedics: a review. J Adv Clin Res Insights 2015;2:94–9.

3. Spolyar JL, Jackson IT, Sullivan W, et al. The Latham technique: Contemporary presurgical orthopedics for the complete oral cleft technique and preliminary evaluation — A bone marker study. Semin Plast Surg 1992;6(1):179–210.

4. Berkowitz S. Neonatal maxillary orthopedics. In: Berkowitz S, editor. Cleft lip and palate, diagnosis and management. 2nd edition. Berlin: Springer; 2005. p. 381–94.

5. Kuijepers-Jagtman AM, Prahl-Andersen B. History of neonatal maxillary orthopedics: past to present. In: Berkowitz S, editor. Cleft lip and palate, diagnosis and management. 2nd edition. Berlin: Springer; 2005. p. 395–407.

6. Spolyar JL. Orthodontics for oral cleft craniofacial disorders. 2nd edition. Philadelphia: Mosby Elsevier; 2010. p. 171–8.

7. Latham RA, Kusy RP, Georgiade NG. An extraorally activated expansion appliance for cleft palate infants. Cleft Palate J 1976;13:253–61.

8. Santiago PE, Schuster LA, Levy-Bercowski D. Management of the alveolar cleft. Clin Plast Surg 2014;41(2):219–32.

9. Weinfeld AB, Hollier LH, Spira M, et al. International trends in the treatment of cleft lip and palate. Clin Plast Surg 2005;32:19–23.

10. Tan S, Greene AK, Mulliken JB. Current surgical management of bilateral cleft lip in North America. Plast Reconstr Surg 2012;129(6):1347–55.

11. Allareddy V, Ross E, Bruun R, et al. Operative and immediate postoperative outcomes of using a Latham-type dentomaxillary appliance in patients with unilateral complete cleft lip and palate. Cleft Palate Craniofac J 2015;52(1):405–10.

12. Millard DR, Berkowitz S, Latham RA, et al. A discussion of presurgical orthodontics in patients with clefts. Cleft Palate J 1988;25(4):403–12.

13. Uzel A, Alparslan ZN. Long-term effects of presurgical infant orthopedics in patients with cleft lip and palate: a systematic review. Cleft Palate Craniofac J 2011;48(5):587–95.

14. Millard DR, Latham R, Huifen X, et al. Cleft lip and palate treated by presurgical orthopedics, gingivoperiosteoplasty, and lip adhesion (POPLA) compared with previous lip adhesion method: a preliminary study of serial dental casts. Plast Reconstr Surg 1999;103(6):1630–44.

15. Latham RA. Bilateral cleft lip and palate: Improved maxillary and dental development. Plast Reconstr Surg 2007;119(1):287–97.

16. Berkowitz S, Meija M, Bystrik A. A comparison of the effects of the Latham–Millard POPLA procedure with a conservative treatment approach on dental occlusion and facial aesthetics in CUCLP and CBCLP. In: Berkowitz S, editor. Cleft lip and palate, diagnosis and management. 2nd edition. Berlin: Springer; 2005. p. 409–49.

17. Costello BJ, Ruiz RL. Cleft lip and palate: comprehensive treatment planning and primary repair. In: Miloro M, editor. Peterson's principles of oral and maxillofacial surgery. 2nd edition. Hamilton (Ontario): BC Decker; 2004. p. 839–58.

18. Fukuyama E, Omura S, Fujita K, et al. Excessive rapid palatal expansion with Latham appliance for distal repositioning of protruded premaxilla in bilateral cleft lip and alveolus. Cleft Palate Craniofac J 2006;52(4):405–10.

19. Kobayashi S, Hirakawa T, Fukawa T, et al. Maxillary growth after maxillary protraction appliance in conjunction with pre-surgical orthopedics, gingivoperiosteoplasty and Furlow palatoplasty for complete bilateral cleft lip and palate patients with protruded premaxilla. Br J Plast Surg 2015;68(6):758–63.

20. Larsen PE. Reconstruction of the alveolar cleft. In: Miloro M, editor. Peterson's principles of oral and maxillofacial surgery. 2nd edition. Hamilton (Ontario): BC Decker; 2004. p. 859–70.

21. Chan KT, Hayes C, Shusterman S, et al. The effects of active infant orthopedics on occlusal relationship in unilateral complete cleft lip and palate. Cleft Palate Craniofac J 2003;40(5):511–7.

Presurgical Dentofacial Orthopedic Management of the Cleft Patient

Kevin S. Smith, DDS[a,b,*], Byron T. Henry, DDS[c,d],
Michelle A. Scott, DDS, MBA[e]

KEYWORDS

- Cleft lip and palate • Dentofacial orthopedic management • Lip taping • DynaCleft
- Grayson-NAM device

KEY POINTS

- Over the last decade, presurgical orthopedic molding for the patient with cleft lip and palate has become much more common; it is even reasonable to assume it may be the standard of care for those wide unilateral and bilateral clefts with substantial dentofacial deformities.
- In 2013, there was a comparative study of nasoalveolar molding methods, comparing the Grayson-NAM device and DynaCleft. The results showed the 2 to be equivocal with both methods significantly reducing the cleft width and improving the nasal asymmetry.
- The lip-taping component of DynaCleft can be used in conjunction with the Grayson-NAM device or can be used with any other maxillofacial orthopedic device.

INTRODUCTION

The cleft lip and palate deformity presents an enormous and complex surgical challenge. Since the earliest reported cleft lip repair in 390 BC, cleft surgeons have continued to strive to perfect this procedure.[1] Cleft lip and palate can arise with considerable variation in form and severity.

Generally speaking, the wider, more extensive clefts are associated with more significant nasolabial deformities, presenting an even greater surgical challenge to obtain functional and esthetic success.[2] Although advances in reconstructive surgery have significantly improved the quality of the repair for clefts of the lip, alveolus, and palate, surgery alone cannot correct all aspects of the defect. The basic goal of any approach to cleft lip, alveolus, and palate is to restore its normal anatomy. Ideally, deficient tissue should be expanded, and malpositioned structures should be repositioned before surgical correction, all allowing for a less invasive surgery to the patient. It is readily agreed on that it is these wide cleft lip and palate cases, wherein alveolar and nasolabial deformities are the greatest, where presurgical noninvasive therapies may be of the most benefit. Presurgical maxillofacial orthopedic treatment appliances address the severe nasolabial deformities, manipulating and minimizing the deformity before surgery and facilitating the repair to improve the surgical outcome.

[a] JW Keys Cleft and Craniofacial Clinic, A Smile for a Child Foundation, University of Oklahoma, Oklahoma City, OK, USA; [b] MK Chapman Cleft and Craniofacial Clinic, University of Tulsa, Tulsa, OK, USA; [c] University of Oklahoma, Oklahoma City, OK, USA; [d] Free to Smile Foundation, Columbus, OH, USA; [e] Nationwide Children's Hospital, Columbus, OH, USA
* Corresponding author. MK Chapman Cleft and Craniofacial Clinic, University of Tulsa, Tulsa, OK.
E-mail address: Kevin-Smith@ouhsc.edu

Oral Maxillofacial Surg Clin N Am 28 (2016) 169–176
http://dx.doi.org/10.1016/j.coms.2016.01.003

HISTORICAL PERSPECTIVE OF MAXILLOFACIAL ORTHOPEDIC THERAPY

Addressing the issues of wide clefts nonsurgically has a history spanning many decades. In 1686, Hoffman described the use of a head cap with extended arms to the face to retract the premaxilla and narrow the cleft.[3]

In 1844, Hullihen stressed the importance of presurgical preparation of clefts using adhesive tape. In 1950, McNeil ushered in the new modern thoughts of presurgical orthopedic treatment in cleft patients with active molding appliances.[4] In 1975, Georgiade and Latham described the intraoral orthopedic device (see Cruz C: Pre-surgical Orthopedics Appliance: The Latham Technique, in this issue) that expanded the collapsed segments while retracting the premaxilla in patients with bilateral cleft lip and palate.[5] One of the problems that the traditional approaches failed to address was the deformity of the nasal cartilages and the columellar tissue deficiency in infants with both unilateral and bilateral cleft lip and palate.[6] Presurgical nasoalveolar molding (PNAM) represented a paradigm shift in thinking from the traditional methods. PNAM was developed by Grayson and colleagues[6] in 1993 with a concept combining an intraoral molding device along with a nasal molding stent. PNAM theory is based on the increased hyaluronic acid in the infant cartilage, lending to the cartilagenous structure having a temporary lack of elasticity and increased pliability and plasticity.[7] The DynaCleft concept was introduced in 2013 as an alternative infant orthopedic device. Also, having both an alveolar component and a nasal component, it adheres to the very same principles as PNAM, recontouring the misshapen deformity and optimizing before surgery. Currently, PNAM is used in many major centers for preoperative orthopedic management of the patient with cleft lip and palate.

OBJECTIVES OF PRESURGICAL DENTAL FACIAL ORTHOPEDICS

The main objectives of PNAM and DynaCleft in patients with unilateral cleft defects are to align and approximate the intraoral alveolar segments and to achieve correction of the nasal cartilages.[6] After completion of the molding, the goal is to have the alveolar segments, nasal cartilages, columella, and philtrum in alignment to facilitate the surgical procedure (**Figs. 1** and **2**). Additional objectives of PNAM in patients presenting with bilateral cleft deformities are to elongate the columella and to reposition the apices of the alar cartilages superior toward the tip. These objectives all serve a single

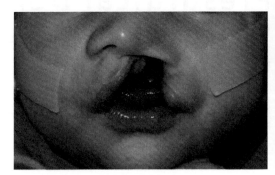

Fig. 1. Unilateral cleft before PNAM.

purpose, to minimize the invasive nature of the surgery, leading to less extensive scarring and an enhanced surgical result.

PRESURGICAL NASOALVEOLAR MOLDING
What Is Presurgical Nasoalveolar Molding?

PNAM is a nonsurgical method to reshape the alveolar segments and nasal tissues before surgery, thus lessening the severity of the cleft defect.

The theory depends on the principles of negative sculpting and passive molding of the alveolus and nasal tissues.[8] Passive molding dictates the growth and direction of the alveolus through custom-made plates. Negative sculpting is a series of modifications to the surface of the molding appliances with the addition or deletion of materials in certain areas to get the desired shape of the alveolus and nose. PNAM takes advantage of the flexibility of the nasal cartilages of the neonate in the first few weeks after birth. This plasticity in the cartilages is caused by the high level of hyaluronic acid found during this time, leaving these cartilages in an optimized state for manipulation.[7] This presenting window of opportunity allows an ease at which external traction and controlled forces can rotate and mold anatomic parts to a more surgically advantageous position.[2] The

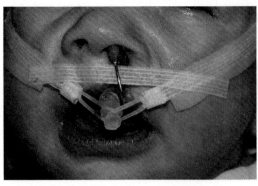

Fig. 2. Unilateral cleft at the end of PNAM.

purpose of this movement is to ultimately lessen the severity of the surgery by facilitating the approximation of the alveolar cleft segments and correcting the nasal cartilage deformity (**Figs. 3** and **4**).

Utilization of the presurgical nasoalveolar molding technique

Introduction and impressions Following complete evaluation and workup by a competent cleft team, the concept of PNAM is explained to the parents of the child, to lessen the anxiety, show them the treatment goals and benefits, and allow them to be involved in the process for their child. The impression of the intraoral cleft defect then follows as early in life as possible, to take advantage of the aforementioned cartilaginous plasticity.[7] A heavy-bodied polyvinyl siloxane impression material is used for the initial impression. The infant is held in an inverted position to keep the tongue forward and to allow fluids to drain out of the oral cavity. It is recommended that this is performed in a hospital setting with facilities to manage any airway emergency and with a surgeon available if needed.[9] Once the impression material has set, the tray is removed, and the mouth is examined for residual material. A nasal impression can also be obtained during this time, even though it is not necessary for PNAM. It is best used to evaluate the preorthopedic and postorthopedic results. The nasal impression is accomplished with a clear polyvinyl siloxane material. The nares are plugged with cotton pellets secured with dental floss to prevent the material from lodging into the nares. After the impression, the cotton pellets are removed, and the nares are inspected for residual material. This impression is then compared with the final result at the end of PNAM.

Device fabrication A model is then prepared using dental stone. The model is duplicated usually as a

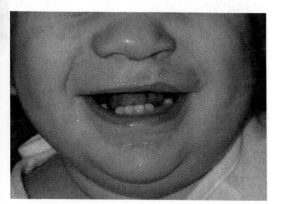

Fig. 3. Six months after lip repair using PNAM.

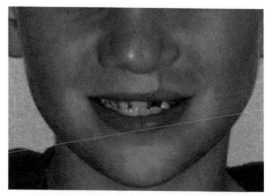

Fig. 4. Six years after lip repair using PNAM.

permanent record to show the changes made after PNAM.

The molding plate is fabricated from a clear methyl methacrylate and is lined with a thin layer of soft denture material. The borders are trimmed, especially in the areas of likely ulceration and the labial frenum area. Its oral portion should be highly polished, and the plate should be fairly retentive with no projections into the cleft area.

Insertion and molding The molding plate is to remain in place full time and only is to be removed for cleaning and routine hygiene practices. Use of a denture adhesive has been described to aid with retention.[10] Immediately after insertion, the child should be observed for retention and proper fit and checked that no acrylic is in the cleft sites. Suckling should be verified, and the presence of gagging needs to be absent. The appliance is secured extraorally to the cheek bilaterally using surgical tape and orthodontic elastics at one end. The elastic loops over a retention arm extending from the anterior flange of the plate at approximately a 40% angle in order to achieve proper activation. The elastic is stretched to twice its original length to achieve the proper activation force of 2 ounces.[2] The direction of elastic pull is in a superior and posterior vector. The surgical tape is best not applied directly onto the skin but rather to a layer of wound care material (Coloplast). The tape is changed once a day. The tape should be applied to the non-cleft side first and then pulled over and adhered to the cleft side.

The patient is followed up weekly to evaluate the molding plate. The plate is evaluated for retention; the intraoral cavity is inspected for possible ulcerations, and the progress of change in the alveolar segments is evaluated for a decrease in the intraoral cleft gap. The molding plate modification is achieved through the selective removal of acrylic from the region into which one desires the alveolar segments to move.

Simultaneously, soft denture-lining material is selectively added to the plate to guide the alveolar segments to a closer approximation, as desired.

In a unilateral patient, the alveolar ridges are guided into a more normal maxillary arch form. In a patient with bilateral cleft, the premaxilla is first derotated, followed by retraction, and the 3 segments are molded to restore a normal maxillary arch alignment.[2] The ideal scenario should have the gingival tissues of the newly repositioned alveolar segments touching.

However, a very successful surgical result may be obtained with a 1- to 2-mm cleft remaining between the segments, or even wider if a gingivoperiosteoplasty is not being performed.[3]

The 1-stage primary cheilorhinoplasty will be performed at 4 to 6 months of age in the patient with unilateral cleft and 6 to 8 months of age in the patient with bilateral cleft. Some surgeons think a gingivoperiosteoplasty is beneficial to perform at the time of lip and nose repair.[11]

Nasal stent When most of the lateromedial correction of the maxillary alveolar segments has been achieved, as evidenced by a reduction in the cleft gap to 5 mm or less and movement of the incisive papilla toward the facial midline, the nasal molding can begin. If this process is started when the gap is too wide, it can lead to an undesirable result in the nares postoperatively that can only be corrected by surgery. The base of the nose and lip alignment is improved with reduction of the alveolar gap.[9] The nasal stent is added to the existing molding plate. The stent is made of stainless steel wire and takes the shape of a "swan neck" that provides access to tape the lip across the cleft.[12] The stent is attached to the labial flange of the molding prosthesis, and a small loop, as described, is created to retain the intranasal hard acrylic component of the nasal stent that is shaped into a bilobed form, resembling the shape of a kidney. A layer of soft denture liner is added to the acrylic for patient comfort and to prevent ulceration to the nasal mucosa.[2] The upper lobe of the bilobed nasal stent is inserted 3 to 4 mm inside the nose and gently lifted forward of the dome until a slight bit of tissue blanching is noted. The lower lobe of the stent lifts the nostril apex and defines the top of the columella. The shapes of the medial and lateral crus, the cartilaginous septum, and the alar cartilage tip are carefully molded to resemble a normal shape by weekly modifications to the nasal stent. Blanching of the nasal tip as the baby suckles and activates the appliance can be observed. Aggressive lip taping is continued after the nasal stent appliance is added.

Nasal stent in the unilateral cleft Only one nasal retentive arm is necessary for the patient with unilateral cleft.

The location of the retentive arm is determined by pulling the cleft lip segments together while centering the columella and philtrum. This junction is marked, and the arm is attached at that location (**Figs. 5** and **6**).

Nasal stent in the bilateral cleft Two retentive arms and 2 nasal stents are necessary for the bilateral cleft. The rationale for the 2 retentive arms is to lengthen the columella. To achieve this, a band of soft denture liner material is added to join the left and right lower lobes of the nasal stents, spanning the columella. The band will sit at the nasolabial junction and defines this angle as the nasal tip continues to be projected forward. Taping continues and is adherent to the horizontal lip tape and is pulled downward to engage the retention arm with elastics. The 2 retentive arms are needed to stabilize the plate on either side of the premaxilla. The 2 nasal stents aid in lifting the nasal ports and creating a counterforce to facilitate stretching the premaxilla. Upward pressure with the nasal stents and downward pull with the premaxilla taping allow the columella tissue stretching. The columella band helps control the vector of the columella stretch (**Figs. 7** and **8**).

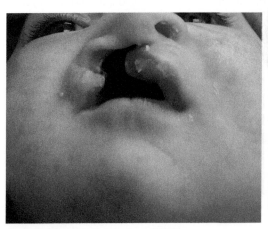

Fig. 5. Unilateral cleft before PNAM.

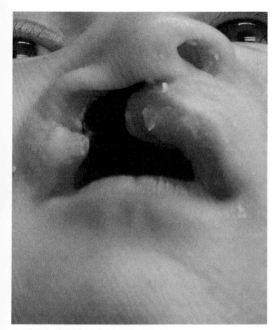

Fig. 6. Unilateral cleft after PNAM.

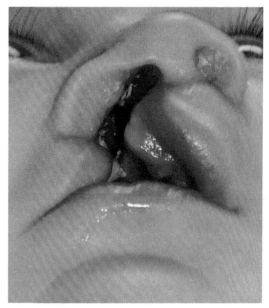

Fig. 8. Bilateral cleft after PNAM.

Benefits of presurgical nasoalveolar molding

The benefits of PNAM are as follows:

- Allows controlled and predictable repositioning of the cleft segments and nasal cartilages without surgery
- Provides reduction in cleft size gap
- Is a one-surgical procedure
- Allows surgeon to perform a gingivoperiosteoplasty, if desired
- Reduces the need for early nasal revision
- Provides columellar elongation in the patient with bilateral cleft

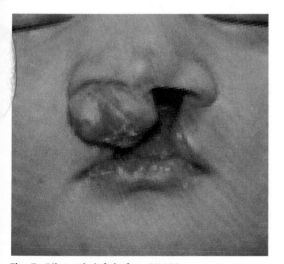

Fig. 7. Bilateral cleft before PNAM.

- Prevents the need for columellar elongation surgery and scar on the orofacial complex of the patient with bilateral cleft
- Improves the infant feeding

Limitations of presurgical nasoalveolar molding

The limitations of PNAM can be listed as follows:

- Compliance of the patient and parents
- Labor intensive
- Weekly visits

Complications of presurgical nasoalveolar molding

The most common complication of PNAM is tissue irritation or ulceration. It is usually due to the taping and skin reaction. Different tapes can be used, and slight adjustments to the location of the tape can be implemented.

Areas of the molding plate may also need to be adjusted as the child's oral cavity is inspected. Overexpansion of the nostril, mega-nostril, is another potential complication of PNAM.[13] Usually the cause is when the nasal stent is applied before the cleft gap is less than 5 mm. Inappropriate vectors of taping can also contribute to this unfortunate complication.

A locked-out segment is another noted complication because of misdirected orthopedic forces. It can be corrected through redirection; yet, additional treatment time is needed, if so. Finally, there is the potential for airway compromise in a situation where the appliance becomes dislodged.

Grayson and Mauli[2] recommend placing a 5-mm hole in the center of the molding appliance so that an air passage is patent should the device drop down onto the tongue and obstruct the airway.

Recent advances in presurgical nasoalveolar molding

Treatment planning and appliance design have recently been described with the use of the CAD technique, enabling accurate analysis of the movement amounts in multiple planes of space.[14] The digital 3-dimensional model of the appliance is constructed using laser scanning to make the diagnosis and measure the movements accurately. A study in 2013 by Yu and colleauges[15] evaluates the effectiveness of CAD-NAM on maxillary alveolar morphology in infants with unilateral cleft lip and palate. The study suggests a trend toward improvements in alveolar repositioning when treated with CAD-NAM.

DYNACLEFT

DynaCleft was introduced and US Food and Drug Administration approved in 2013 as an alternative to the Grayson-NAM device in presurgical orthopedic alveolar movements. It was developed in conjunction with cleft teams and uses tape with an elastomeric core to bridge the cleft segments, gently guiding tissue and bone into a better surgical position. The principle of passive molding, as noted in the PNAM concept, is used to allow the cleft segment repositioning. After applied appropriately to the infant, the tension from the elastomeric band distributes over the misshapen alveolar cleft segments, placing a vector of appropriate force to manipulate the segment into its more normal anatomic position. DynaCleft has tape for both a unilateral (DCX-10) and a bilateral (DCX-20) cleft deformity (**Fig. 9**). DynaCleft also has a nasal component as well, focusing solely to reshape the nasal cartilaginous structures. The theory is similar to what is described in the PNAM section of nasal cartilage molding.

DynaCleft Tape Application

Unilateral has a cleft and non-cleft side to the taping band. The larger portion of the elastic tape is adapted to the cleft side.

Bilateral has a central portion that should be positioned on the premaxilla with care to avoid the junction of the columella and prolabium to avoid soft tissue ulcerations (**Fig. 10**).

DynaCleft elastomeric tape bands should be replaced every 2 days, to compensate for elastic fatigue and to allow further molding with appropriate forces.

Nasal Component of DynaCleft

The nasal stent component is hook shaped. It is positioned just inside the nares toward the nasal septum and suspended by a skin-friendly adhesive band that is placed on the patient's forehead. The force of suspension of the hook should be such that slight blanching is noted on the alar rim. Too much pressure or blanching may result in necrosis or ulceration of the nasal skin and mucosa. Like the elastic lip bands, the nasal stent should be replaced every 2 days as well, as the cartilage continues to remodel and needs adjustment.

Benefits of DynaCleft

The benefits of DynaCleft can be listed as follows:

- Is less labor intensive and has decreased treatment cost when compared with other orthopedic molding devices
- Repositions the cleft segments and nasal cartilages without surgery (**Fig. 11**)

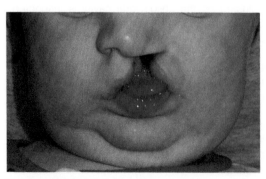

Fig. 9. Unilateral cleft lip before surgery.

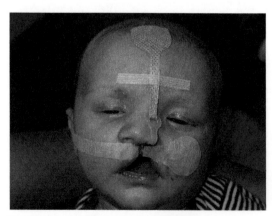

Fig. 10. DynaCleft lip and nasal taping.

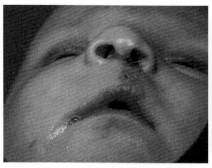
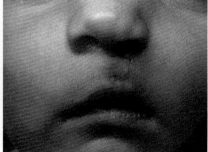

Fig. 11. Immediately postoperatively after DynaCleft use.

- Reduces in cleft size gap
- Is one surgical procedure
- Reduces the need for early nasal revision
- Improves the infant feeding

Limitations of DynaCleft

The limitations of DynaCleft can be listed as follows:

- Does not allow columellar elongation in the patient with bilateral cleft
- Allows compliance of the patient and parents
- Requires periodic visits for adjustments of the nasal stents

Complications of DynaCleft

The most common complication of DynaCleft is dermatitis and ulceration of the cheeks (**Fig. 12**). This complication is usually due to skin reaction to the adhesive on the tape and is generally observed less frequently in the DynaCleft tape compared with use of traditional Steri-Strips. Overexpansion of the nostril or misdirection of nasal stent placement can result in inappropriate nasal cartilage molding.

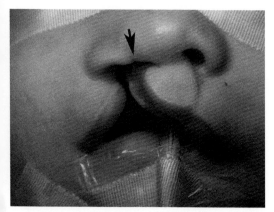

Fig. 12. Notching of the lower lateral cartilage of the nares after using the DynaCleft nasal stent.

A locked-out premaxillary segment can also occur because DynaCleft does not allow for any expansion of the lateral alveolar ridges in a patient with bilateral cleft. Last, the elastic tape band may break during its use.

SUMMARY

In 2013, there was a comparative study of nasoalveolar molding methods, comparing the Grayson-NAM device and DynaCleft.[15,16] The results showed the 2 to be equivocal, with both methods significantly reducing the cleft width and improving the nasal asymmetry. The lip-taping component of DynaCleft can be used in conjunction with the Grayson-NAM device or can be used with any other maxillofacial orthopedic device. DynaCleft requires less frequent recall and adjustment visits, has a lower overall treatment fee, and may offer some advantages for those patients living very far away and without financial means.

Over the last decade, presurgical orthopedic molding for the patient with cleft lip and palate has become much more common. It is even reasonable to assume it may be the standard of care for those wide unilateral and bilateral clefts with substantial dentofacial deformities. As noted, PNAM and DynaCleft both have roles in the treatment of these patients. Certainly, as the research continues and the potential of this modality of treatment in helping these cleft deformities continues to be discovered, their applications will become even more prevalent.

REFERENCES

1. Wu LT. Wong, history of Chinese medicine. Shanghai (China): Mercury Press; 1936.
2. Grayson BH, Mauli D. Nasoalveolar molding for infants born with clefts of the lip, alveolus, and palate. Clin Plast Surg 2004;31:148.
3. Smith KS. Presurgical orthopedic management of the cleft patient. In: Turvey TA, editor. Oral and

maxillofacial surgery. Chapter 38. 2nd edition; 2009. p. 783–90.

4. Grayson BH, Shetye PR, Cutting CB. Presurgical nasoalveolar molding treatment in the cleft lip and palate patients. Colin J 2005;1:4–7.

5. Gorgiade N, Latham R. Maxillary arch alignment in the bilateral cleft lip and palate infant, using pinned coaxial screw appliance. Plast Reconstr Surg 1975; 56:52.

6. Grayson BH, Santiago PE, Brecht LE, et al. Presurgical nasoalveolar molding in infants with cleft lip and palate. Cleft Palate Craniofac J 1999;36:486.

7. Matsuo K, Hirose T, Otagiri T, et al. Repair of cleft lip with nonsurgical correction of nasal deformity in the early neonatal period. Plast Reconstr Surg 1989;83: 25–31.

8. Habel A, Sell D. Management of cleft lip and palate. Arch Dis Child 1996;74:360–4.

9. Brecht LE, Grayson BH, Cutting CB. Nasolaveolar molding in early management of the cleft lip and palate. In: Taylor TD, editor. Clinical maxillofacial prosthetics. Chicago: Quintessence; 2000. p. 63–84.

10. Ezzat CF, Chavarria C, Teichgraeber JF, et al. Presurgical nasoalveolar molding therapy for the treatment of the unilateral cleft lip and palate: a preliminary study. Cleft Palate Craniofac J 2007;44:8.

11. Millard DR, Latham RA. Improved primary surgical and dental treatment of clefts. Plast Reconstr Surg 1990;86:856.

12. Doruk C, Kilic B. Extraoral nasal molding in a newborn with unilateral cleft lip and palate: a case report. Cleft Palate Craniofac J 2005;42:699–702.

13. Taylor T. Complications associated with pre surgical nasoalveolar molding and columellar lengthening. Clinical Maxillofacial Prosthodontics; 2015.

14. Gong X, Yu Q. Correction of maxillary deformity in infants with bilateral cleft lip and palate using computer-assisted design. Oral Surg Oral Med Oral Pathol Oral Radiol 2012;114(Suppl 5):s74–8.

15. Yu Q, Gong X, Shen G. CAD presurgical nasoalveolar molding effects on maxillary morphology in infants with UCLP. Oral Surg Oral Med Oral Pathol Oral Radiol 2013;116:418–26.

16. Monasterio L, Ford A, Gutierrez C, et al. Comparative study of nasoalveolar molding methods: nasal elevator plus DynaCleft versus NAM-Grayson in patients with complete unilateral cleft lip and palate. Cleft Palate Craniofac J 2013;50(5):548–54.

Otologic Concerns for Cleft Lip and Palate Patient

Wayne Berryhill, MD

KEYWORDS

- Middle ear dysfunction • Cleft lip and palate • Ear tubes

KEY POINTS

- Cleft palate is associated with greater than a 90% persistence of middle ear fluid (OME) and management with pressure equalization tubes.
- Middle ear dysfunction is caused by clefts.
- Frequent audiologic assessment and ORL assessment is necessary to limit the impact of cleft palate–associated eustachian tube dysfunction.

Understanding eustachian tube physiology and anticipating probable eustachian tube dysfunction is an important component of cleft palate management. This article provides a brief summary of the otologic physiology and issues that may be of concern to cleft palate management. It is of critical importance not only to provide primary closure of the cleft palate, but to also recognize that along with speech, hearing has a critical component to the educational and social success of all individuals.

It is common for children with cleft palate to suffer from eustachian tube dysfunction and ensuing sequela. This dysfunction leads to negative pressure within the middle ear space, associated quiescent serous or mucoid otitis media, infectious acute otitis media, and then chronic otitis media as a progression of conditions. In the absence of intervention, repeated cycles of infection place the tympanic membrane under severe positive and negative pressure, leading to atrophy or scarring of the tympanic membrane. It is essential to involve audiology and otorhinolaryngology in the assessment and care of these children to ensure best hearing conditions possible. Best hearing conditions are achieved with a normal tympanic membrane under neutral pressure with normal ossicular chain.

The human eustachian tube is an organ system comprised of a cartilaginous skeleton, peritubal muscles, mucosal lumen, and osseous component and associated Ostmann fat pad. The purpose of the eustachian tube organ system is to provide optimal sound pressure transfer conditions to the inner ear by ventilation of pressure within the middle ear and mastoid space, middle ear protection, and the clearance of middle ear secretions.

Bluestone and Klein[1] in 1972 described the differences between the infant and adult eustachian tube. Adult eustachian tube characteristics are achieved by 18 years of development and growth. The infant eustachian tube begins at a length of 14 to 19 mm and reaches full length between 31 and 38 mm by the age of 7. The angle of the infant eustachian tube is 10° from horizontal and changes by elongation and anterior progression of mid-face development to 45° from horizontal in the adult. Cartilage density increases through growth and development, and increase in size of Ostmann fat pad. Elastin and mucosal folds decrease over time.

The eustachian tube begins at the anterior superior middle ear space as an osseous ovoid opening and passes anteriorly, medially, and inferiorly through the petrous temporal bone with the tensor

Oklahoma Otolaryngology Associates, 3650 West Rock Creek Rd, Norman, OK 73072, USA
E-mail address: wayne.berryhill@gmail.com

Oral Maxillofacial Surg Clin N Am 28 (2016) 177–179
http://dx.doi.org/10.1016/j.coms.2015.12.001
1042-3699/16/$ – see front matter © 2016 Elsevier Inc. All rights reserved.

tympani and carotid artery as companion medial boundaries. The osseous portion of the eustachian tube is normally patent and lined with mucous-producing cells and ciliated cells and represents approximately a third of the total eustachian tube distance. Passing along a gentle curved course anteriorly and inferiorly the osseous lumen incorporates into the cartilaginous lumen.

The cartilaginous ligament is closed in a resting position with mucosal lumen. The cartilage is intimately attached to the skull base and is classically described as an inverted "J." The lateral short portion of the inverted "J" is relatively constant in height, and in the medial long arm increases its height as it approaches its attachment to the medial pterygoid plate.[2] It is lined with ciliated pseudostratified columnar epithelium. The cartilage portion of the eustachian tube continues its anterior and inferior curved descent to the opening in the nasopharynx known as the torus tubarius. The proportions and dimensions of the eustachian tube show great variability for size and course.[3]

The classic description of the union of the osseous and cartilaginous portions of the eustachian tube is that of two cones connected at their narrow necks, in a region known as the isthmus. The isthmus corresponds to the region of the bony cartilaginous junction. The lower cone, corresponding to the cartilaginous portion, is collapsed at rest and does not allow nasopharyngeal fluid to egress up the tube, providing the protective function of the eustachian tube. The lateral membranous wall of the tube is comprised of fibrous tissue and paratubal muscle insertions.

The eustachian tube muscles are comprised of the tensor veli palatine, levator veli palatine (LVP), salpingopharyngeus, and the tensor tympani. The tensor veli palatini provides active opening of the eustachian tube. The tensor veli palatine arises from the base of the medial pterygoid plate and the lateral wall of the eustachian tube and forms a tendon around the hamulus of the medial pterygoid plate to insert into the palatine aponeurosis. The LVP arises from the apex of the petrous portion of the temporal bone and from the medial wall of the eustachian tube and inserts into the palatine aponeurosis. The LVP acts as a dilator of the cartilage. The salpingopharyngeus acts as a very minor depressor of the floor of the tube and arises from the medial and inferior tube to join the palatopharyngeal muscle mass.

These muscles work in concert to open the valve region of the eustachian tube during swallowing, yawning, crying, and sneezing. Adequate opening of the tube allows equalization of the pressure within the middle ear to that of the atmosphere.

Failure of eustachian tube opening and adequate equalization leads to the accumulation and presence of negative pressure within the middle ear space. Lack of equalization and inadequate opening impede the clearance function of the eustachian tube via the mucociliary system and the stasis of middle ear and mastoid fluid. Negative pressure and/or the presence of fluid stasis are optimal conditions for otitis media.

Cleft palate is associated with greater than a 90% persistence of middle ear fluid (otitis media with effusion [OME]) and management with pressure equalization tubes.[4] The presence and persistence of fluid and the likely near-term inability to establish eustachian function lead to the near universal recommendation that these children receive pressure equalization tubes to prevent otologic complications. The timing of myringotomy and tube placement should be individualized to the specific patient with abnormal physical examination and testing. Patient medical conditions, external auditory canal size, planned surgical procedures, number of acute otitis media, and abnormal tympanograms assist in determining the appropriate timing of intervention. OME does not allow normal function of the middle ear and causes a 25- to 40-dB hearing loss.[5] Early onset hearing loss is associated with speech development delay, language impairment, and decreased cognitive ability.[6,7] Acute otitis media is a positive pressure process causing the bulging of the tympanic membrane. Cycles of acute otitis media followed by OME can lead to atrophy of the tympanic membrane or scarring of the membrane, known as tympanosclerosis. Atrophic membranes are prone to rupture and collapse into the middle ear space. Repeated infection alters the mucosa of the middle ear and mastoid. Retraction of atrophic tympanic membranes can cause damage to underlying ossicles, erosion of ossicles, and adhesion of the tympanic membrane to abnormal mucosa of the middle ear, worsening conductive hearing loss. For these reasons frequent audiologic assessment and otorhinolaryngology (ORL) assessment is necessary to limit the impact of cleft palate–associated eustachian tube dysfunction.

REFERENCES

1. Bluestone CD, Klein JO. Otitis media in infants and children. 2nd edition. Philadelphia: WB Saunders; 1995.
2. Matsune S, Sando I, Takahashi H. Abnormalities of lateralcartilaginous lamina and lumen of Eustachian tube in cases of cleft palate. Ann Otol Rhinol Laryngol 1991;100:909.

3. Swarts JD, Rood SR, Doyle WJ. The fetal development of the auditory tube and paratubal musculature. Cleft Palate J 1986;23:289.

4. Muntz HR. An overview of middle ear disease in cleft palate children. Facial Plast Surg 1993;9(3):177–80.

5. Hunter LL, Margolis RH, Giebank GS. Identification of hearing loss in children with otitis media. Ann Otol Rhinol Laryngol 1994;163:59–61.

6. Ruben RJ, Bagger-Sjoback D, Chase C. Complications and sequelae. Ann Otol Rhinol Laryngol 1994; 103(Suppl 164):67–80.

7. Teele DW, Klein JO, Rosner BA, The Greater Boston Otitis Media Study Group. Otitis media with effusion during the first three years of life and development of speech and language. Pediatrics 1984;74(2): 282–7.

Diagnosis and Management of Velopharyngeal Dysfunction

Robert S. Glade, MD, FAAP[a,b,*], Randolph Deal, PhD[c]

KEYWORDS

- Velopharyngeal dysfunction • Velopharyngeal insufficiency • VPI • VPD • Nasoendoscopy
- Nasopharyngoscopy • Videofluoroscopy • Palatoplasty

KEY POINTS

- Velopharyngeal dysfunction (VPD) describes any condition whereby the velopharyngeal valve does not properly close during the production of oral sounds, with multiple causes, including velopharyngeal mislearning (nasopharyngeal sound substitution for an oral sound), velopharyngeal incompetence (neurolophysiologic dysfunction causing poor pharyngeal movement), and velopharyngeal insufficiency (a structural or anatomic defect prevents velopharyngeal closure).
- Evaluation for VPD is best performed within the context of a multidisciplinary team and consists of history and physical examination, perceptual speech evaluation, and instrumental assessment of speech with either video nasoendoscopy or multiview speech fluoroscopy.
- Speech therapy is the mainstay in treatment of velopharyngeal mislearning, while velopharyngeal inadequacy and insufficiency may require surgical intervention after a trial of speech therapy.
- Surgical correction of VPD is based on the size and location of the velopharyngeal gap seen during instrumental assessment and includes posterior wall augmentation, Furlow palatoplasty, sphincter pharyngoplasty, and pharyngeal flap.

 Video content accompanies this article at http://www.oralmaxsurgery.theclinics.com/

INTRODUCTION

With the exception of /m/, /n/, and /ng/, all phonemes within the English language are produced orally and require complete or nearly complete closure of the velopharyngeal mechanism to be perceived as normal. If air or sound is allowed to leak through or resonate in the nasal chamber during production of the nonnasal sounds, speech will be marked by hypernasal resonance and nasal air emission.

ANATOMY

It is generally agreed that 3 muscles contribute to velopharyngeal closure. The levator veli palatini is a paired muscle that originates on the inferior surface of the temporal bone near the torus tubarius (where the eustachian tube exits the temporal bone) and along the medial lamina of the eustachian tube cartilage. The fibers course downward and forward, intertwining with fibers of the superior constrictor muscle in the lateral nasopharyngeal wall. They ultimately insert into the velum at a 45° angle where they meet the contralateral fibers. Most of the fiber pairs are found in the mid one-third of the velum, where they form a slinglike structure. When contracted, levator pulls the velum up and back against the posterior nasopharyngeal wall (above the level of the atlas) while also

[a] Oromaxillofacial Surgery, Oklahoma University, Oklahoma City, OK, USA; [b] Otolaryngology–Head and Neck Surgery, Oklahoma State University, Tulsa, OK, USA; [c] University of Oklahoma Health Sciences Center, Oklahoma City, OK, USA
* Corresponding author. Pediatric ENT of Oklahoma, 10914 Hefner Pointe Drive, Suite 200, Oklahoma City, OK 73120.
E-mail address: rglade@peds-ent.com

Oral Maxillofacial Surg Clin N Am 28 (2016) 181–188
http://dx.doi.org/10.1016/j.coms.2015.12.004
1042-3699/16/$ – see front matter © 2016 Elsevier Inc. All rights reserved.

collapsing the side walls of the nasopharynx medially. In this manner, the entire velopharyngeal port can be closed. The sphincter complex of the superior constrictor is paired and originates at the pharyngeal raphe. Its fibers course forward and medially to enter the velum from either side. On contraction, the sphincter complex acts as a pseudosphincter and can close the velopharyngeal port circumference. In some patients, the posterior pharyngeal wall is pulled anteriorly by this muscle complex, creating an anterior bulging of the posterior pharyngeal wall during velopharyngeal closure. This phenomenon is called Passavant pad (Video 1). Curiously, sometimes it occurs too low in the posterior pharyngeal wall to aid velopharyngeal closure during speech. Finally, muscularis uvula is paired and originates on either side of the posterior nasal spine. The fibers course posteriorly, approaching the velum. On contraction, they add thickness to the posterior third of the velum, helping to occlude the velopharyngeal port.

TERMINOLOGY

Several terms have been used interchangeably to describe the multiple causes responsible for inappropriate airflow through the nasopharynx during speech; this has led to redundancy and confusion in both medical literature and communication between practitioners. In this article, the following commonly accepted definitions are used. Velopharyngeal dysfunction (VPD) describes any condition in which the velopharyngeal valve does not close completely and consistently during the production of oral sounds. VPD has multiple causes, which are broadly grouped into 3 distinct subgroups based on root cause (**Fig. 1**). These causes include velopharyngeal mislearning (VPM), velopharyngeal incompetence, and velopharyngeal insufficiency (VPI). VPM describes the creation of certain sounds within the nasopharynx as a substitution for oral sounds. This behavior is learned, with no anatomic or neurophysiologic source. Velopharyngeal incompetence refers to a neurophysiologic disorder resulting in poor velopharyngeal movement. Palatal structure and anatomy are normal, including length, but poor movement prevents complete closure of the velopharyngeal valve. VPI describes a structural or anatomic defect that prevents closure of the velopharyngeal mechanism, such as overt or submucous cleft palate.

Distinguishing the precise cause of VPM is essential, because the treatment of VPM, velopharyngeal insufficiency, and VPI varies.

CAUSE

The most common cause of VPI is children with an overt cleft palate. Despite successful palatoplasty, the incidence of VPI after surgery has been reported to be as high as 20% to 50%.[1,2] VPI is also seen in submucous cleft palate, where no overt cleft is seen, but the levator muscle fibers fail to fuse in the midline. These VPIs classically manifest with the triad of a bifid uvula, diastases in the midline (caused by insertion of the levator muscles onto the hard palate rather than into a midline raphe), and hard palate notch. Interestingly, many children with submucous cleft will have no evidence of VPI during their lifetime, and management is only required when symptoms exist.[3] In an occult submucous cleft palate, similar to submucous cleft palate, the levator muscles insert onto the posterior hard palate but a bifid uvula or midline diastasis is not present.[4] Occult submucous cleft palate is best diagnosed by video nasopharyngoscopy, where a sagittal orientation of the levator muscles is noted with an absence of the muscularis uvulae (Video 2). VPI is rarely

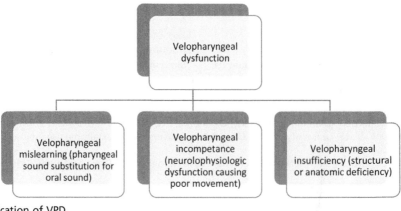

Fig. 1. Classification of VPD.

seen after adenoidectomy, but is more likely to occur if a submucous cleft is present and not diagnosed. In fact, in reviews of children noted to have VPI after adenoidectomy, 26% to 55% were noted to have a previously undiagnosed submucosal cleft palate.[5,6] In rare cases, tonsillar hypertrophy may restrict velopharyngeal closure, causing VPI, which is alleviated after tonsillectomy (Videos 3 and 4).

VPD in the absence of anatomic or structural dysfunction is also seen. In this scenario, it is often secondary to velopharyngeal incompetence. Causes consist of many neurologic disorders, including posttraumatic brain injury, cerebral palsy, myasthenia gravis, multiple sclerosis, Parkinson disease. In a recent study by Goudy and colleagues,[7] 44% of patients with VPD without cleft palate were diagnosed with a velopharyngeal mechanism suffering from neurologic dysfunction. Also, several syndromes may manifest with VPI with or without cleft palate. Most commonly, velocardiofacial syndrome (VCFS), an autosomal-dominant disorder linked to microdeletions in the long arm of chromosome 22, has a very large spectrum of phenotypes and often includes facial dysmorphisms, cardiac anomalies, and VPD. Although overt and submucous cleft palate may be seen in VCFS, hypotonia of the velopharyngeal mechanism is common and may lead to VPD despite no cleft. VPD is also a common feature in Kabuki syndrome, which shares many features with those of VCFS. Other syndromes in which VPD has been noted include trisomy 21, Klippel-Feil, epidermal-nevus syndrome, Alagille syndrome, Turner syndrome, and VATER (vertebral anomalies, anal atresia, tracheoesophageal fistula, esophageal atresia, radial and renal anomalies).[7,8]

DIAGNOSIS

Assessment of VPD is most accurately performed through evaluation within the context of a multidisciplinary team, which includes a VPD surgeon, an experienced speech and language pathologist (SLP), and an otolaryngologist. A detailed patient history and physical examination are required in addition to perceptual speech examination and instrumental assessment of the velopharyngeal mechanism. Instrumental assessments include video nasoendoscopy (VNE) and multiview speech video fluoroscopy (MSVF).

The patient history should include questions examining whether a comorbid condition is present, history of a syndrome, history of cleft palate, whether nasal regurgitation while feeding is also present, and a history of recurrent ear infections. It is critical to obtain a detailed sleep history,

including the presence of snoring, restless sleep, and witnessed apneas. A detailed history from the patient's primary speech therapist may also be beneficial.

During physical examination, otoscopy of the tympanic membrane often will reveal otitis media with effusion or retraction of the drum, indicating eustachian tube dysfunction; this is commonplace among children with VPI. Oropharyngeal examination is focused on the entire soft palate, including movement; tonsils; and teeth, including occlusion. Children with symptoms of sleep-disordered breathing often require a polysomnogram before intervention. As discussed earlier, tonsillar hypertrophy may inhibit palatal closure and may be a source of VPI. If obstructive sleep apnea or tonsillar hypertrophy is present, it is generally accepted that it should be addressed before surgical management of VPD, which potentially worsens symptoms by narrowing an already obstructed airway.

PERCEPTUAL SPEECH EVALUATION

A perceptual speech evaluation should be performed by an SLP with experience in diagnosis and treatment of children with VPD. In the authors' multidisciplinary clinic, the following assessment is performed.

Excessive Nasal Resonance (Hypernasality)

To rule out possible confounding effects of an obstructed nasal airway on excessive nasal resonance, a nasal patency test is performed. This look-and-listen test involves first observing whether the patient is mouth breathing. If so, it is important to determine whether the mouth breathing observed is due to an obstructed airway. Mouth breathing can be habitual. With the patient's lips closed, evaluation for excessive nasal air flow stridency, bilaterally and unilaterally by alternately occluding each nare during exhalation, is noted. This evaluation can also be assessed by placing a mirror under the nares and observing the fogging pattern. Adequate nasal air flow is characterized by circles about the size of a quarter. Mouth breathing in the presence of reasonable nasal patency is likely habitual.

Assuming a patent nasal airway, a nasal pinch test is performed. The patient is asked to sustain a high vowel, for example, /ʊ/ or /ɪ/ (which requires complete velopharyngeal closure). Although the patient sustains the vowel, the clinician alternates pinching and not pinching the nares. If velopharyngeal closure is adequate, there will be no change in the sound quality between the pinch and no-pinch conditions (no cul-de-sac resonance during the pinch), and the inference is adequate velopharyngeal valve closure. However, if during the pinch, cul-de-sac resonance is heard, the clinician cannot necessarily assume an incompetent velopharyngeal valve, because some patients lower the velum when the nares are pinched.

Next, the severity of the perceived oral-nasal resonance imbalance is judged to infer velopharyngeal status for speech. This judgment can be done using a variety of equal-appearing intervals scales of severity (usually 5, 7, or 9 point scales) or a direct magnitude estimation scale. One clinically useful scale might be 1 = normal; 2 = mild hypernasality; 3 = moderate hypernasality, and 4 = severe hypernasality. Conversational speech, prepared sentences, word lists, or isolated sustained vowels can be used as samples to judge. Regardless, because resonance is being judged, the clinician should focus on the voiced components of the sample and whether excessive nasal resonance is perceived on phonemes other than the nasals. Speech stimuli loaded with vowels and glides (/w/, /r/, /l/, for example) would be particularly helpful in isolating the hypernasality from the other manifestations of velopharyngeal inadequacy.

Audible Nasal Emission

When the velopharyngeal valve is inadequate, audible nasal emission of air during speech sounds requiring the buildup of intraoral pressure is typically present; this can be perceived in conversational speech, sentences, and word lists. Therefore, although plosives, fricatives, and affricates all require high intraoral pressure, voiceless fricatives require complete, sustained velopharyngeal closure. One particularly high demand on the velopharyngeal mechanism is the counting sequence from 60 to 70. The word, "sixty," for example, is composed of a voiceless fricative /σ/, then a high vowel /l/, followed by a triple cluster (voiceless plosive, voiceless fricative, voiceless plosive) /κστ/, then a high vowel /ι/. If a patient presents VPI, counting from 60 to 70 becomes nearly impossible without revealing speech manifestations related to VPI, for example, audible nasal emission, hypernasality, and/or speech misarticulations.

Speech Misarticulations Related to Velopharyngeal Insufficiency

Typically, SLPs use one of many available standardized articulation tests to examine the articulation of the various consonants and vowels. These tests require the patient to produce common, short words that have the test phoneme in the initial, medial, and final positions of words. For example, words for the test phoneme /π/ would

include pictures of pig, puppy, and cup. The clinician shows the picture to the patient and asks, "What's that?"; or the words can be imitated by the patient from the clinician's request, "Say ___." Sentences containing words loaded with the test phoneme can also be read or repeated by the patient. However, accurate and reliable recording of the patient responses takes practice.

During the evaluation, the SLP should be able to draw some tentative conclusions regarding whether the patient's speech is indicative of VPD. For example, normal dialectical nasality will present with oral-nasal resonance imbalance but typically will not manifest either audible nasal emission of air or misarticulations related to VPI. Also, the presence of glottal stop substitutions or phoneme-specific nasal emission of air (usually on /σ/) is sometimes seen in children with otherwise normally developing speech articulation and normal nasal resonance. Perceived nasality associated with VPI, however, will more likely present all.

Video Nasoendoscopy

VNE allows for direct visualization of the velopharynx during speech. It is performed by inserting a small, flexible fiberoptic laryngoscope through a nasal cavity anesthetized with topical lidocaine and decongested with oxymetazalone. The view is enhanced by passing the scope through the middle meatus instead of along the nasal floor in order to look down on the velopharyngeal mechanism. From above, the endoscopist is able to visualize closure of the soft palate, lateral pharyngeal wall movement, orientation of the levator veli palatini, and any gaps during speech that may be present. Observation of a "groove" on the central nasal surface of the soft palate indicates a sagittal orientation of the levator veli palatini muscle,[9] indicative of a submucous cleft palate (see Video 2).

The major limitation of this study is that younger patients often have difficulty cooperating with the examination, which requires production of and extended speech sample with the scope present in the nasal cavity. It is the authors' experience that typically around the age of 6, most children are able to fully cooperate; however, they have had success with many children as young as 4 years of age. Another limitation is that quantitatively measuring anatomic findings including gap size is difficult. Standardized reporting techniques exist, however, making estimations possible.[10]

Various closure patterns may be noted on VNE, which are mainly dependent on movement of the levator veli palatini and superior constrictor, creating lateral wall movement, and occasional posterior pharyngeal wall muscle constriction. Variations of 4 different closure patterns are typically described (**Fig. 2**).

Multiview Speech Video Fluoroscopy

Before improvements in pediatric sized flexible laryngoscopes offered images with excellent resolution, multiview fluoroscopy was the mainstay for assessment of the velopharyngeal mechanism in children. It is still used as the primary instrumental assessment of VPD in many centers and is performed as a collaborative effort between a radiologist and SLP. Typically, after a small amount of high-density barium is injected via syringe into a child's nose to coat the nasopharynx, 3 radiographic views are obtained while an SLP guides the patient through a standard speech sample. An anterior-posterior view allows excellent assessment of lateral pharyngeal wall motion and a lateral view allows visualization of movement of the soft palate and the posterior pharyngeal wall. A base view allows visualization of the sphincter as a whole. This study is an excellent alternative for children who do not tolerate VNE.

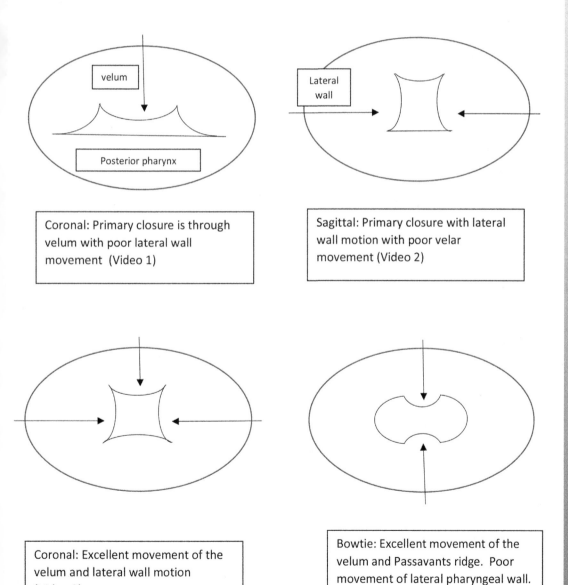

Coronal: Primary closure is through velum with poor lateral wall movement (Video 1)

Sagittal: Primary closure with lateral wall motion with poor velar movement (Video 2)

Coronal: Excellent movement of the velum and lateral wall motion (Video 3)

Bowtie: Excellent movement of the velum and Passavants ridge. Poor movement of lateral pharyngeal wall.

Fig. 2. Closure patterns seen on VNE.

Disadvantages include exposing children to ionizing radiation and compliance with younger children. It is also very difficult to assess postsurgical findings, especially in the setting of a pharyngeal flap.

Even though the size of velopharyngeal gap is more objectively assessed by instrumental assessment versus perceptual speech evaluation, they can still only estimate gap size. Multiple articles have compared the advantages and disadvantages of VNE to MSVS; however, superiority of one has not been clearly established. A review by Lam and colleagues[11] revealed that each modality may provide complementary data, but VNE may provide a higher correlation with VPI severity. Currently, it is the authors' practice to perform VNE to assist surgical planning on all patients and will limit MSVF for children who do not tolerate VNE or where additional information after a VNE is required.

Nasometry

Nasometry measures the amount of nasal acoustic energy relative to nasal plus oral acoustic energy in a person's speech. The ratio is expressed as a percentage and is termed "nasalance." Nasalance is performed with a headset attached to a sound separator, which is placed between the nose and the upper lip. Microphones are carried by the separator and are oriented directly in front of the nose and the mouth. The microphones can then differentiate between oral and nasal signals, and these are compared with normative values. Preoperative and postoperative nasalance scores may be compared to assess surgical success.

TREATMENT
Nonsurgical

Speech therapy is the mainstay in treatment of children with VPM. It is also essential to treat compensatory misarticulations, which have resulted from VPI. It is important that speech therapy continue after surgical correction of an anatomic defect when these misarticulations exist.

Dental appliances are usually poorly tolerated by children, but can be used as temporary treatment or for poor surgical candidates. These devices are custom-made by a prosthodontist and designed to anchor into the maxillary dentition similar to a retainer. A palatal lift is designed to elevate a soft palate with adequate length that is unable to contact the posterior pharyngeal wall secondary to neurogenic dysfunction. It contains posterior extensions that lift the soft palate superiorly. An obturator is designed to fill the open gap between the soft palate and posterior pharyngeal wall when palatal length is insufficient.[12]

Surgical Management

Surgical management is typically the first line of treatment for VPI. Multiple techniques have been described to treat the defects created by different closure patterns. Controversy exists as to the merits and relative efficacy of each. These procedures include, but are not limited to, posterior wall augmentation (including injection pharyngoplasty), Furlow palatoplasty, sphincter pharyngoplasty, and pharyngeal flap. It is the authors' practice to tailor the procedure based on the size and location of the anatomic defect.

Posterior Wall Augmentation

Posterior wall augmentation involves placing material within the posterior pharyngeal wall, causing its anterior displacement and effectively creating "a speed bump," which narrows the distance that the soft palate must travel in order to obtain contact. Multiple injectable materials have been used in the past, including fact, fascia, acellular dermis, and calcium hydroxylapatite. The authors use the technique described by Sipp and colleagues,[13] in which the calcium hydroxylapatite is injected under direct visualization using a 120° telescope. The authors have found this technique to be especially effective in VPI noted after adenoidectomy in children without overt cleft palate. In general, this technique is best used on the child with a small, central, velopharyngeal gap and mild VPI.

Furlow Palatoplasty (Double Opposing Z-plasty)

The Furlow palatoplasty was initially designed as a treatment for primary cleft palate repair. Its elegant design not only closes a soft palate defect but also provides a means to lengthen the palate by reorienting the direction of the levator veli palatini muscles into a transverse orientation. It is a mainstay in the treatment of both submucous and occult submucous cleft palate.[14] Multiple studies have shown that it can be effectively used as a secondary treatment for VPI after primary cleft palate repair.[15–17] Success of this technique is dependent on careful patient selection and has been correlated with small velopharyngeal gaps estimated to be less than 5 mm to 1 cm in depth.[15,18,19] Also, it should be reserved for palates that are both kinetic and show a sagittal orientation of the levator muscles. Its principal advantage is that patients have a lower risk of developing obstructive sleep apnea than with both sphincter pharyngoplasty and pharyngeal flap.[20]

Sphincter Pharyngoplasty

The sphincter pharyngoplasty was first introduced by Hynes[21] in 1950. Although several modifications of his original procedure have been introduced through the years, the general concept remains unchanged.[22,23] It involves creating 2 superior based flaps from the region of the posterior tonsillar pillars (which may or may not include the palatopharyngeus muscles). These flaps are rotated 90° into a transverse incision made high in the posterior pharyngeal wall mucosa. The flaps may be sutured end to end or overlapped, thus giving the surgeon control over the amount of narrowing of the resultant velopharyngeal port. Theoretically, this dynamic flap is placed in an orientation that creates a dynamic sphincter as well as a "speed bump" on the posterior pharyngeal wall. A postoperative study using video fluoroscopy suggests that the sphincter may exhibit some degree of dynamics.[24] By rotating the lateral pharyngeal walls medially, sphincter pharyngoplasty is generally used in the setting of a child with a sagittal or bowtie closure pattern (poor lateral pharyngeal wall movement with adequate movement of velum) (Video 5). Its success is dependent on adequate function of the velum, which must close the central port during speech production.

Pharyngeal Flap

Schoenborn introduced the first pharyngeal flap procedure in 1875. In his initial description, an inferiorly placed flap created from the posterior pharyngeal wall was inserted into the soft palate. Later, he described the first superior based flap in 1886.[25,26] Since that time, multiple variations of this procedure have been described, but the general principle remains the same. Tissue from the posterior pharyngeal wall is raised and secured into the soft palate (via both splitting and not the soft palate), effectively creating a permanent obturator in the central nasopharynx. This obturator significantly decreases airflow through the velopharyngeal port. Nasal patency is preserved through 2 ports on the lateral sides of the flap (Video 6). Success of the procedure is dependent on adequate lateral pharyngeal wall movement during speech, which obturates the ports and obstructs airflow through the nasopharynx during speech.[27] This procedure should be most effective for patients with a sagittal or circular closure pattern with adequate lateral wall motion.

Table 1
Ideal patient for surgical correction of velopharyngeal insufficiency

Surgical Procedure	Ideal Patient
Posterior wall augmentation	Small central gap, postadenoidectomy VPI
Furlow palatoplasty	Submucous, occult submucous cleft palate, and secondary cleft palate repair with small gap (<5 mm to 1 cm) (see Video 2)
Sphincter pharyngoplasty	Coronal or bowtie closure pattern with lateral gaps (see Video 5)
Pharyngeal flap	Sagittal or central closure pattern with large, central gap, inadequate palatal length, palatal hypotonia (Video 7)

SUMMARY

Evaluation of VPD is complex and is best performed within the context of a multidisciplinary team. Evaluation should involve both perceptual speech examination by an experienced SLP and an instrumental assessment of VPI with either VNE or MSVF. Surgery is the mainstay for VPI with procedure selection based on size and location of gap (**Table 1**).

SUPPLEMENTARY DATA

Supplementary data related to this article can be found online at http://dx.doi.org/10.1016/j.coms. 2015.12.004.

REFERENCES

1. Kummer AW. Anatomy and physiology: the orofacial structures and velopharyngeal valve, cleft palate and craniofacial anomalies, the effects on speech and resonance. San Diego (CA): Singular; 2001. p. 3–32.
2. Morris HL. Velopharyngeal competence and primary cleft palate surgery, 1960-1971; a critical review. Cleft Palate J 1973;10:62–71.
3. McWilliams BJ. Submucous clefts of the palate: how likely are they to be symptomatic? Cleft Palate Craniofac J 1991;28:247–9 [discussion: 250–1].
4. Kaplan EN. The occult submucous cleft palate. Cleft Palate J 1975;12:356–68.

5. Trier WC. Velopharyngeal Incompetence in the absence of overt cleft palate: anatomic and surgical considerations. Cleft Palate J 1983;20:209–17.

6. Shpritzen RJ, Golberg RB, Lewin ML, et al. A new syndrome involving cleft palate, cardiac anomalies, typical facies, and learning disabilities. Cleft Palate J 1978;15:56–62.

7. Goudy S, Ingraham C, Canady J. Noncleft velopharyngeal insufficiency: etiology and need for surgical treatment. Int J Otolaryngol 2012;2012:296073.

8. Kallen B, Mastroiacovo P, Robert E. Major congenital malformations in Down syndrome. Am J Med Genet 1996;65(2):160–6.

9. Rudnick EF, Sie KC. Velopharyngeal insufficiency: current concepts in diagnosis and management. Curr Opin Otolaryngol Head Neck Surg 2008; 16(6):530–5.

10. Golding-Kushner KF, Argamaso RV, Cotton RT, et al. Standardization for the reporting of nasopharyngoscopy and multiview video fluoroscopy: a report from an International Working Group. Cleft Palate J 1990;27(4):337–47.

11. Lam DJ, Starr JR, Perkins JA. A comparison of nasoendoscopy and multiview videofluoroscopy in assessing velopharyngeal insufficiency. Otolaryngol Head Neck Surg 2006;134:394–402.

12. Willging JP. Velopharyngeal insufficiency. Curr Opin Otolaryngol Head Neck Surg 2003;11:452–5.

13. Sipp JA, Ashland J, Hartnick CJ. Injection pharyngoplasty with calcium hydroxyapatite for treatment of velopalatal insufficiency. Arch Otolaryngol Head Neck Surg 2008;134(3):268–71.

14. Chen PK, Wu J, Hung KF, et al. Surgical correction of submucous cleft palate with Furlow palatoplasty. Plast Reconstr Surg 1996;97(6):1136–46.

15. Chen PK, Wu JTJ, Chen YR, et al. Correction of secondary velopharyngeal insufficiency in the cleft palate patients with the Furlow palatoplasty. Plast Recontstr Surg 1994;94(7):933–41.

16. Perkins JA, Lewis CW, Gruss JS, et al. Furlow palatoplasty for management of velopharyngeal insufficiency; a prospective study of 148 consecutive patients. Plast Reconstr Surg 2005;116(1):72–80.

17. Sie KC, Tampakopoulou DA, Sorom J, et al. Results with Furlow palatoplasty in management of velopharyngeal insufficiency. Plast Reconstr Surg 2001; 108(1):17–25.

18. D'Antonio LL, Eichenberg BJ, Zimmerman GJ. Radiographic and aerodynamic measures of velopharyngeal anatomy and function following Furlow Z-plasty. Plast Reconstr Surg 2000;106(3):539–49.

19. Deren O, Ayhan M, Tuncel A. The correction of velopharyngeal insufficiency by Furlow palatoplasty in patients older than 3 years undergoing Veau-Vardill-Kilner palatoplasty: a prospective clinical study. Plast Reconstr Surg 2005;116(1):85–93.

20. Liao YF, Noordhoff MS, Huang CS, et al. Comparison of obstructive sleep apnea syndrome in children with cleft palate following Furlow palatoplasty of pharyngeal flap for velopharyngeal insufficiency. Cleft Palate Craniofac J 2004;41(2):152–6.

21. Hynes W. Pharyngoplasty by muscle transplantation. Br J Plast Surg 1950;3(2):128–35.

22. Hynes W. The results of pharyngoplasty by muscle transplantation in failed cleft palate cases, with special reference to the influence of the pharynx on voice production; Hunterian lecture, 1953. Ann R Coll Surg Engl 1953;13(1):17–35.

23. Orticochea M. Construction of a dynamic sphincter in cleft palates. Plast Reconstr Surg 1968;41(4):323–7.

24. Witt PD, Marsh JL, Arlis H, et al. Quantification of dynamic velopharyngeal port excursion following sphincter pharyngoplasty. Plast Reconstr Surg 1998;101:1205–11.

25. Passavant G. Ueber die Beseitgung der Naselnden Sprache bei angeborenen Spalten des harten und weichen Gaumens. Arch Klin Chir 1865;6:333–49.

26. Schoenborn D. Vorstellung eines Falles staphyloplastik. Verhandlungen der Deutschen Gesellschaft fur Chirurgie 1886;15:57.

27. Argamaso RV, Shprintzen RJ, Strauch B. The role of lateral pharyngeal wall movement in pharyngeal flap surgery. Plast Reconstr Surg 1980;66(2):214–9.

Rhinoplasty for the Cleft Lip and Palate Patient

Angelo Cuzalina, MD, DDS[a],*, Calvin Jung, MD, DDS[b]

KEYWORDS

- Cleft rhinoplasty • Secondary rhinoplasty • Nasal revision • Unilateral cleft deformity

KEY POINTS

- Definitive rhinoplasty is a complex surgery given the anatomy and surrounding tissue bed due to previous surgeries.
- Rib cartilage provides structural support and ample supply of cartilage for the multiple areas that require grafting.
- Deficiencies at the piriform rim and premaxilla require augmentation to improve symmetry of the nasal sill.

INTRODUCTION

Cleft rhinoplasties are regarded as a very challenging surgery to perform. The reasons are numerous but are mainly due to the architectural deformity of the cartilage, skeleton, or skin (primary), or scarring of the surrounding tissue bed from previous surgeries (secondary). The range of the deformity can be mild to severe and has a causal relationship to the degree of lip deformity.[1]

A search of the literature reveals numerous surgical techniques that have been advocated to repair the cleft nasal deformity. Contemporary craniofacial surgeons have focused on the importance of primary rhinoplasties, with or without nasoalveolar molding devices, followed by secondary, definitive, rhinoplasties. This article touches on both techniques; however, the focus is based on the authors' experiences and techniques for the secondary, or definitive, rhinoplasty.

CLEFT NASAL DEFORMITY ANATOMY
Unilateral Cleft Deformity

The characteristic defects that are present in patients with a unilateral nasal cleft are listed in Box 1. These characteristics have been well documented and consistent.[1,2] The hallmark of a unilateral cleft deformity is a 3-dimensional asymmetry involving the nasal tip and alar base. Discontinuity of the orbicularis oris on the cleft side and improper insertion into the columella on the noncleft side will produce an unopposed pull of the columella and caudal septum in the direction of the noncleft side[3] (**Fig. 1**). On the cleft side, the insertion of the orbicularis to the alae produces an effect on the alar base, pulling it laterally, inferiorly and posteriorly.[4,5]

The asymmetry with the nasal tip on the cleft side is due to a short medial crus and long lateral crus compared with the medial and lateral crus of the noncleft lower lateral cartilage (LLC). The vector of muscle pull and asymmetric LLC will produce a nostril that is wide and horizontally oriented.[6,7] The nasal septum will deviate toward the noncleft side caudally and the septum will deflect toward the cleft side posteriorly (**Fig. 2**).

Bilateral Cleft Nasal Deformity

The nasal deformity of a bilateral cleft is grossly symmetric and shares many features found in a

Disclosure Statement: The authors have nothing to disclose.
[a] Private Practice Tulsa Surgical Arts, 7322 East 91st Street, Tulsa, OK 74133, USA; [b] Private Practice, Premier Surgical Arts, 2024 Richmond Avenue, Houston, TX 77098, USA
* Corresponding author.
E-mail address: angelo@tulsasurgicalarts.com

Oral Maxillofacial Surg Clin N Am 28 (2016) 189–202
http://dx.doi.org/10.1016/j.coms.2015.12.002
1042-3699/16/$ – see front matter © 2016 Elsevier Inc. All rights reserved.

unilateral cleft deformity[1,3] (see **Box 1**). The major features include short columella with a wide base, lack of nasal tip definition, and alar bases that are caudally and laterally positioned. The lateral crus of the LLC is longer in bilateral clefts that, combined with short medial crus, will lead to

underprojection of the nasal tip and caudal, lateral, and inferior positioning of the alar bases (**Fig. 3**). The nasal septum is classically midline; however, if gross asymmetry exists, the septum will deviate toward the less affected side.[8,9] It should be noted that, due to poor cartilage structure and support, the external valves, as well as the internal nasal valves, can be affected, leading to potential nasal breathing difficulties.[10]

SURGICAL TIMING
Primary Cleft Rhinoplasty

This article primarily focuses on the authors' treatment of secondary, definitive, rhinoplasties. However, treatment of the cleft nose at the time of initial cleft lip intervention is now increasingly accepted and the positive effects on secondary rhinoplasties have been well documented. Initial reservations with primary rhinoplasties were based on the principle that manipulation of the surrounding tissue bed would create adverse scarring and affect growth centers of the nose. Multiple investigators have dispelled this notion.[11]

The primary goal of this procedure is the closure of the nasal floor, symmetric repositioning of the LLC, and repositioning of the alar base.[12] The addition of nasoalveolar molding device in conjunction with the primary surgery has been advocated because there is an improvement in alar base symmetry and lengthening of the columella.[11,13]

Definitive Cleft Rhinoplasty

Definitive rhinoplasties are performed at the conclusion of nasal or maxillary growth. Most cleft patients also have midface hypoplasia requiring maxillary repositioning with a Le Fort 1 osteotomy. If the cleft patient requires orthognathic surgery, the rhinoplasty is often performed after the skeletal discrepancies have been addressed. In male patients, the optimal age for definitive rhinoplasty is between 16 and 18 years old. For female patients, it is between 14 and 16 years old. These surgical procedures allow for improved projection of the maxilla without affecting the dorsum.[14] The effects of orthognathic surgery will allow for anterior movement of LLC and improving tip projection.

Septum

As discussed previously, the septum deviates toward the noncleft side, bowing away from the nasal spine (see **Fig. 1**). Resection of this portion of the septum allows for correction of the deviated portion of the septum[15] and care is given to leave at least 10 mm L-strut (dorsum and caudal) for

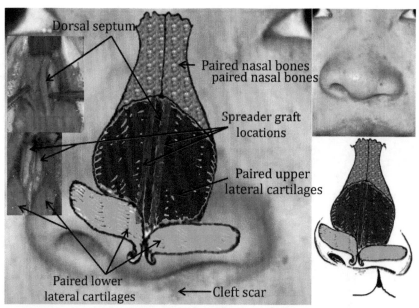

Fig. 1. Classic nasal aesthetic issues for a patient with a unilateral cleft lip and palate. Paired upper lateral cartilages (*blue*) have asymmetric caudal (inferior) elongation of the cartilage on the cleft side. The paired lower lateral cartilages (*green*) have move severe asymmetric changes on the side of the cleft resulting in both caudal decent of the ala and horizontal widening of the ala on the side of the cleft from a frontal view. The areas of the internal nasal valve (adjacent the septum and upper lateral cartilages) is commonly treated with spreader grafts (*red*). Although these are common in revision nasal surgery, grafts such as batten-type onlay grafts are much more often indicated in the cleft palate patient to correct external nasal issues.

support in most cases. However, some cases of deviation are so severe that more can be removed as long as a straight piece is replaced to give support that would otherwise be lost. Often, removal of the deviated portion of the septum cannot relieve the residual memory left in the L-strut (**Fig. 4**). The L-strut often remains deviated and sutures placed through the upper lateral cartilages

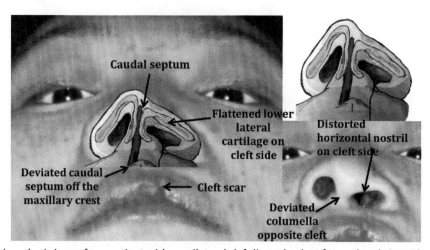

Fig. 2. Nasal aesthetic issues for a patient with a unilateral cleft lip and palate from a basal view. The paired LLCs (*green*) have move severe asymmetric changes on the side of the cleft, resulting in sometimes extremely severe flattening of the ala and horizontal widening of the ala on the side of the cleft. The condition is compounded by the bony deficiency along the piriform rim on the cleft side. Inadequate improvement of a cleft patient's rhinoplasty is common if the surgeon addresses only cartilage issues and fails to augment the piriform rim on the cleft side. Further asymmetry can be see if the caudal septum (*red*) is deflective to the side of the maxillary crest.

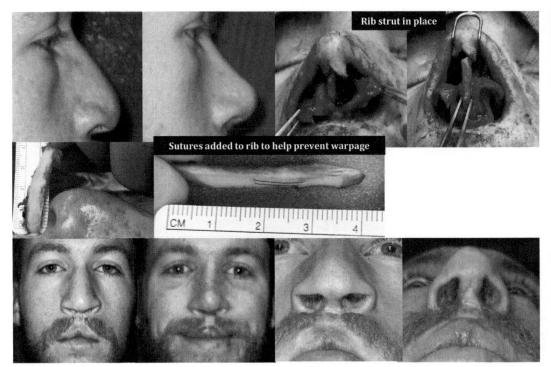

Fig. 3. 21-year-old male patient with bilateral cleft lip and palate before and 2 years following rhinoplasty using rib cartilage as a septal extension graft. A curved rib cartilage was used for large batten onlay grafts, plus left piriform onlay rim grafting using thick cartilage and screw fixation. The patient also required cephalic cartilage strip excision, tip suturing, and lateral osteotomies to narrow the nose.

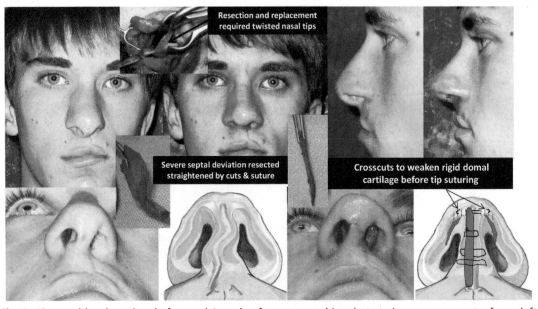

Fig. 4. 19-year-old male patient before and 4 weeks after an open rhinoplasty to improve asymmetry from cleft and a severely deviated caudal septum. Cephalic strip cartilage excision was performed on lower lateral crural cartilages. A large strut from the septum (straightened with crosscuts and suture) was placed along with trans-domal suturing after crosscuts are made at the dome to narrow the tip and increase tip projection. The caudal septum was trimmed to treat the hanging columella and the medial crura sutured to the residual septum more cephalically.

(ULCs) and septum that apply a vector in the opposite direction of the deviation are placed to help correct the asymmetry **Fig. 5**. Other techniques that can aid in straightening of the septum involve using robust spreader grafts as struts along the dorsal margins and surgical repositioning of the caudal septum[16,17] (see **Fig. 1**). By repositioning the remnant of the caudal septum from the deviated position to the midline allows for alignment of the septum to the nasal final point. This realignment is technically accomplished by suture fixation of the caudal portion of the L-strut to the nasal spine. Some surgeons advocate placing a notch in the nasal spine and using it as an additional support layer to which the septum can be sutured. If there is residual memory in the cartilage after it has been set into the nasal spine, it can be alleviated by scoring the cartilage.

The resected portion of quadrangular cartilage serves as an excellent reservoir to use for spreader grafts or batten grafting. Care is taken to preserve the curvatures within the deviated septum and to use each piece to the advantage of the natural curves of the nose. For example, if a surgeon were to graft the dorsum of the nose, it would allow the convexity of the septal cartilage to be placed facing the skin envelope (**Fig. 6**). This would prevent the cartilage from warp or flex. Access to the quadrangular cartilage is readily available when performing the definitive rhinoplasty via an open incision. Dissection is carried between the medial crura of the LLC to gain access to the septum. Care must be taken when developing a mucoperichondrial flap to not perforate or damage the surrounding mucosa. This will allow for meticulous access and surgical precision.

Spreader Grafts

Spreader grafts are easily used because they are harvested from the resected deviated septal cartilage or from sectioned pieces of rib cartilage. Spreader grafts are placed between the septum and ULCs to repair collapsed internal nasal valves and improve airflow. The spreader grafts can also be used to help straighten and keep the septum midline. The caudal end of the graft can serve as a strut to which extension grafts to aid in tip support can be sutured or manipulated (see **Fig. 1**).

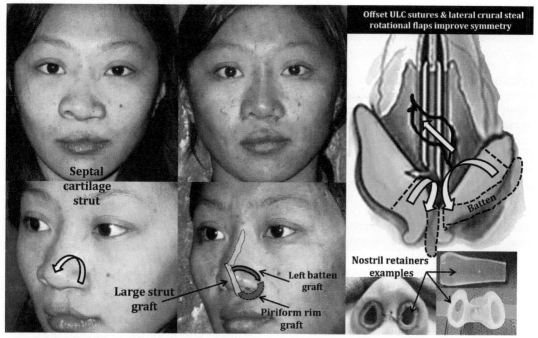

Fig. 5. 18-year-old Chinese female patient before and 6 months following open rhinoplasty plus permanent lip augmentation to improve symmetry and appearance due to a left unilateral cleft lip and palate. She is nearly identical to the patient in **Fig. 4**. However, due to more severe tip ptosis and poor tip strength, rib cartilage was the ideal choice for graft material. To increase projection, a thick midline strut was attached to the caudal septum and lateral crural medialized flaps. The asymmetry was improved with a batten graft and piriform rim graft on the left using rib and offset sutures in the ULCs (*blue*). An alar crease Weir-type incision was used for access to the piriform rim and nostril restructuring on the left with alar base narrowing. Nostril retainers for 1 week helped maintain ideal nasal form during early postoperative edema. *Yellow arrows* are indicating the vector of movement of the cartilage and vector of force of suture.

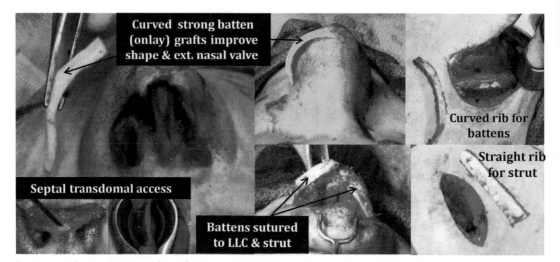

Fig. 6. Use of curved pieces of cartilage, specifically rib cartilage, as long and sturdy batten onlay grafts. The external nasal valve is reinforced to allow much improved breathing. The paired LLCs (*green*) have move severe asymmetric changes on the side of the cleft, resulting in caudal decent of the ala and horizontal widening of the ala on the side of the cleft from a frontal view. ext, external.

Dorsum or Nasal Osteotomies

The dorsum deviates away from the cleft and is typically wide and asymmetric. In cleft patients, the nasal dorsum is also flat and underprojected. The authors' preferred method for correction of this deficiency is with either a silicone implant or a carefully carved piece of rib cartilage as a dorsal onlay graft (**Figs. 7** and **8**).

Abnormalities in the nasal bones are common and, as with the septum, often deviate toward the noncleft side. Also prevalent in cleft patients with a dorsal hump, isolated removal of the dorsal hump without addressing other facets of the nose will lead to unsymmetrical changes, mainly a severe open-roof deformity. The dorsal hump peaks at the rhinion where the ULC and nasal bones join. Reduction of the dorsal hump is aided by rasping of the nasal bones and reduction of the ULCs via scissors or blade. Lateral osteotomies are performed to help narrow the width and create symmetry. Some cleft patients with wide nasal dorsa will also require medial osteotomies to aid in aesthetics. An osteotomy is performed with a small osteotome along the planned osteotomy. The most common techniques are sliding osteotomy with a Neivert osteotome or a micropuncture technique with a small osteotome. Both techniques have advantages and disadvantages. The authors prefer to use a 2 to 3 mm osteotome and perform micropunctures along the planned osteotomy (see **Fig. 7**).

Nasal Tip or Lower Lateral Cartilages

Many techniques have been advocated for manipulation and modifications of the LLCs. From the profile view (see **Fig. 8**; **Fig. 9**), it can be appreciated that the tip is blunted with an arched alae. The LLC on the cleft side is also caudally displaced and flat. Most cleft patients have similar features that require surgical intervention to correct. Access to the LLCs through an open rhinoplasty incision aids in manipulation and correcting differences in the LLCs. Excision of small cephalic strips of LLCs can be performed as required to narrow a bulbous nasal tip and improve symmetry via removal of more on the larger side (see **Fig. 7**). Once removed, transdomal dissection to expose the caudal septum is performed and deviation corrected by resection and replacement. A strong septal extension graft can be added to aid in tip support and improve projection[14,18] (**Fig. 10**). The cartilage can rotate an acute nasolabial angle from a ptotic nasal tip back to a normal angle. The strut (extension graft) can be sutured between the dome of the LLC and the caudal portion of the septum, as well as be secured to spreader grafts if used. Spreader grafts are used if there is evidence of internal valve collapse (positive Cottle test) preoperatively or if the surgery itself may cause problematic narrowing of the valve. The base of the nose can be strengthened by bolster sutures of the medial crus to the septal cartilage graft.

To further establish symmetry and additional tip projection, lateral crural advancement flaps (lateral crural steal) are used (**Fig. 11**). The vertical length of the medial crus of the LLC is shorter on the cleft side, whereas the lateral crus is longer and more horizontal than the noncleft side. With an elongated and asymmetric LLC that is short in vertical height, it is advantageous to lengthen the LLC on

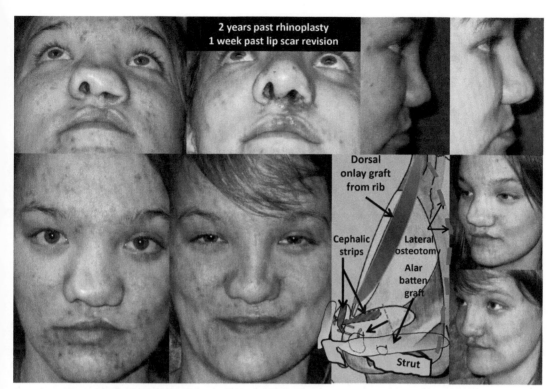

Fig. 7. 19-year-old female patient before and 2 years following rhinoplasty as well as a lip scar revision to improve symmetry and appearance due to a left unilateral cleft lip and palate, and an underdeveloped midnasal region, resulting in a saddle nose deformity. Rib cartilage was harvested for a septal extension graft, large batten grafts, L > R, dorsal onlay graft, left piriform onlay rim graft, and lateral crural advancements. The patient also had minor cephalic cartilage strip excision. The wide saddle nose deformity and severe tip ptosis with no support must be adequately addressed.

the cleft side via the lateral crural steal approach. This allows for improved symmetry of the tip by using the longer crural flap on the cleft side to increase projection of the tip on that side. Reconstruction of the lateral crura is competed by robust cartilage struts or batten grafts that can be place below the residual lateral crus or above as onlay type grafts (see **Figs. 5, 6** and **9**). Finally, further tip projection can require a shield graft that can improve symmetry as well as projection and tip shape (see **Fig. 9**).

The tissue bed at the tip of the nose requires that the cartilage graft provide enough structural support to improve tip support but also resist the resulting scar tissue that will form in this region. A minimum of 4 to 5 cm long septal extension graft that is a least 1 mm thick should be placed to allow for improved projection and resist deprojection from the surrounding tissue (see **Figs. 8** and **10**). Septal cartilage is readily available because there are no additional incisions required and no additional donor site morbidity. The use of septal cartilage also allows for simultaneous correction of septal deviations. The use of rib cartilage in

definitive rhinoplasties is common given the abundance of cartilage available that can be manipulated for multiple regional deficiencies. The use of rib graft as a septal extension allows for maximal strength to resist postinflammatory changes (see **Fig. 3**). Rib cartilage also allows the surgeon to have extra cartilage that is often needed for other areas of the cleft patient's nose.

Piriform Rim and Premaxilla Augmentation

The nasal sill is often missing or severely deficient (**Fig. 12**). From the base view, this deficiency can be appreciated. Additionally, the skeletal deficiencies in the premaxilla lead to posterior and inferior displacement of the skeletal unit on the cleft region. Augmentation of this specific area will help to improve projection and symmetry; whereas ignoring the boney deficiency will almost guarantee that the final result will be less symmetric than desired. When a rib graft has been harvested, a portion of the graft can be used for piriform rim augmentation (see **Fig. 12; Fig. 13**). Stacking of cartilage will aid in improving anterior

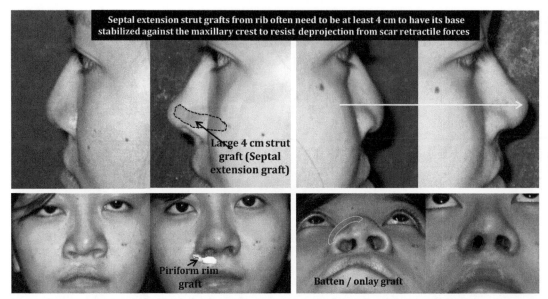

Fig. 8. 17-year-old Vietnamese female patient before and 1 month following open rhinoplasty plus permanent lip augmentation to improve symmetry and appearance due to a right unilateral cleft lip and palate. To increase projection, a sturdy strut from rib also known as a septal extension graft, was attached to the caudal septum and lateral crural medialized flaps. The asymmetry was improved with a batten graft and piriform rim graft on the right using rib. The septal extension graft requires a longer length in cleft patients because of scar retraction that is more powerful than in noncleft patients. 4 to 5 cm long strut with adequate thickness better resists deprojection, particularly if the inside end rests securely against bone and resists rotation by multiple sutures attaching it to caudal septum and dome cartilages.

projection. Alternatively, if rib cartilage is not used, a silicone piriform rim implant can be used.

Alar Base Reduction

At the completion of the rhinoplasty, addressing the nasal alae is often the final step. Most cleft alae are laterally and inferiorly displaced (see **Figs. 5, 7** and **8**). Two techniques that have been described to fix this asymmetry are the Weir procedure and V-Y advancement along the alar facial groove.[19–21] However, true symmetry will also require cleft-sided nostril vertical enlargement

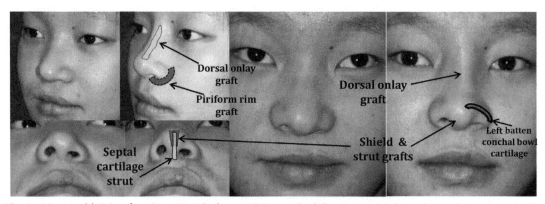

Fig. 9. 14-year-old Asian female patient before and 6 months following open rhinoplasty plus permanent lip augmentation to improve symmetry and appearance due to a left unilateral cleft lip and palate. Septal and ear cartilage was harvested instead of than rib because the deformity was relatively mild and the patient was having a simultaneous otoplasty. To increase projection, a septal midline strut was used in combination with a conchal shield graft in the tip. The asymmetry was improved with a batten graft on the left from conchal cartilage and stacked septal cartilage along the left piriform rim. Small cephalic strips and tip suturing with 5-0 polydioxanone suture suture helped narrow the tip in addition to the strut. Further improvement likely would have been achieved with left superior nostril skin resection or flap rotation but was not performed.

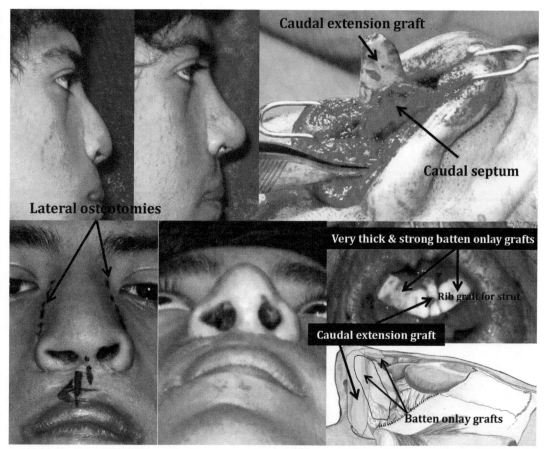

Fig. 10. 24-year-old Hispanic male patient with bilateral cleft lip and palate before and 1 year following rhinoplasty using rib cartilage used for a septal extension graft. Curved rib cartilage was used to create 2 large batten onlay grafts. The patient also required cephalic cartilage strip excision, tip suturing, and lateral osteotomies to narrow his nose.

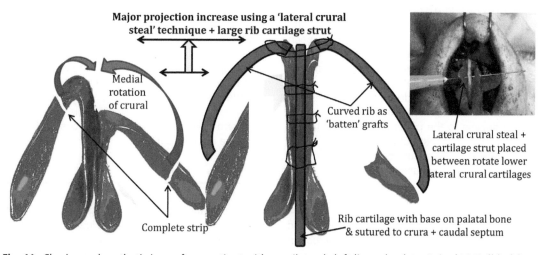

Fig. 11. Classic nasal aesthetic issues for a patient with a unilateral cleft lip and palate. Paired ULCs (*blue*) have asymmetric caudal (inferior) elongation of the cartilage on the cleft side. The paired LLCs (*green*) have move severe asymmetric changes on the side of the cleft, resulting in caudal decent of the ala and horizontal widening of the ala on the side of the cleft from a frontal view.

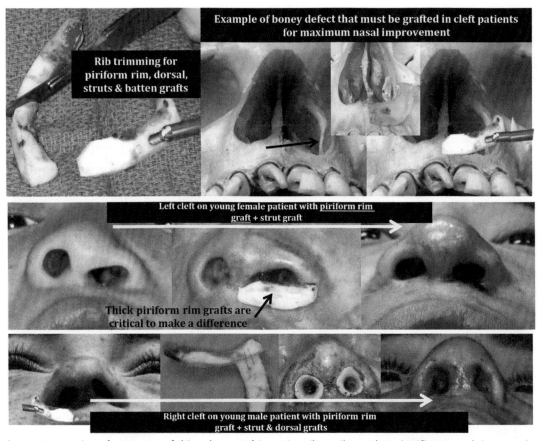

Fig. 12. Progression of treatment of rhinoplasty grafting using rib cartilage when significant nasal tip retraction and asymmetry exist. Due to scarring and major bone, as well as cartilage abnormalities, cleft lip and palate patients require most aggressive treatment to obtain a stable result for many years. *Black arrow*, shows the deficiency of bone on that left side of the patient vs the right.

and rim augmentation in addition to the common 2 alar type reductions[22] (see **Fig. 13**). When the nostril itself is not addressed, the result can still be excellent except from the basal view in which the nostril vertical height discrepancy can be seen (**Fig. 14**). For lateral skin excess, the Weir procedure (alar resection) is the authors' preferred method for improving the symmetry of the alar base in which the cleft-side nostril is longer and elongated.[23–26] Using the Weir procedure also allows for access to the piriform rim for grafting in addition to alar base restructuring. Nostril retainers (see **Figs. 5** and **12**) are sutured into place to help maintain and mold the nasal sill.

Rib Cartilage

Autologous tissue is always preferred to alloplastic implants given the higher incidence of infection and potential dehiscence for synthetic materials in the nose. When a patient presents with a severe lack of nasal projection, and septal cartilage is insufficient and larger quantities of cartilage are needed, rib cartilage is an excellent source. Additionally rib cartilage is robust and sturdy, allowing it to resist scar contracture and provide excellent support for improving nasal projection. The advantages of rib cartilage are numerous, including ample supply of cartilage for grafting; versatility with respect to shape, size, and width; and rigidity and support. The disadvantages of rib cartilage include warpage of the graft, extra morbidity of a secondary donor site, external visible scar, pneumothorax, postoperative pain, and ossification of cartilage in older patients.

Technique

It is the authors' preference to harvest cartilage from the patient's right side. Digital palpation of the sternomanubrial joint will indicate the position of the second rib. Palpation is now taken inferiorly to, and harvest will be from, the sixth or seventh rib (**Fig. 15**). Once the area has been marked, an incision is made through the skin using a 10 blade and dissection is made through subcutaneous tissue,

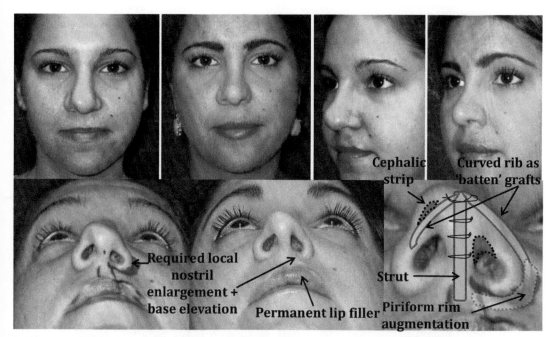

Fig. 13. 27-year-old female patient before and 2 years following rhinoplasty plus permanent lip augmentation to improve symmetry and appearance due to a left unilateral cleft lip and palate. Rib cartilage was harvested to create a large and sturdy midline strut to increase projection, a large batten grafts, L > R, plus left piriform onlay rim grafting using thick cartilage and screw fixation. The patient also required right cephalic cartilage strip excision and an inward skin flap of the superior edge of the left ala to help match the height of the nostrils.

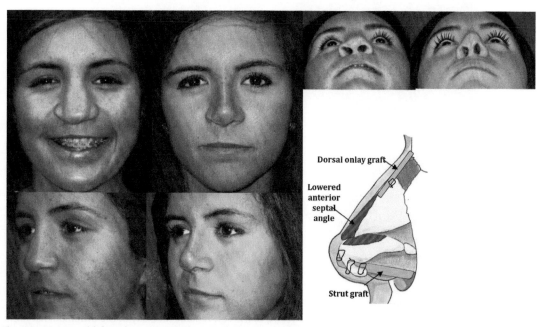

Fig. 14. 16-year-old female patient before and 18 months following rhinoplasty plus permanent lip augmentation to improve symmetry and appearance due to a left unilateral cleft lip and palate. Rib cartilage was harvested to create a large and sturdy midline strut to increase projection, a large batten graft, R > L, plus left piriform onlay rim grafting using thick cartilage and screw fixation. The patient also required right cephalic cartilage strip excision and an inward skin flap of the superior edge of the left ala to help match the height of the nostrils.

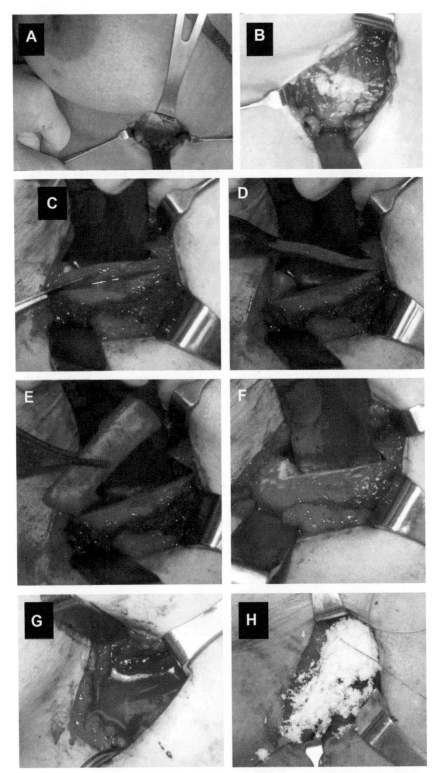

Fig. 15. Harvesting right sixth or seventh rib cartilage. (*A*, *B*) Incision is made medially in the inframammary fold and dissection exposes the cartilaginous portion of the rib with the most ideally shaped cartilage. (*C–F*) Subperichondrial elevation is carefully performed around the rib and a malleable retractor used to prevent lung injury during resection of required cartilage shape and volume. (*G*) Positive pressure via anesthesia with saline in the site verifies no pneumothorax. (*H*) Avitene or other collagen matrix helps prevent a hematoma when placed before closure.

muscle, and fascial using an electrocautery instrument. Once the rib is visualized, care is taken to make an incision in the center of the rib to incise through the perichondrium. Dissection should be carried medially to the junction of the sternum and cartilage, and laterally to the osseous cartilaginous junction in a subperichondrial plane. The dissection is continued to the posterior portion and a retractor is placed posterior to the rib to protect from inadvertent injury to the perichondrium. Once the medial and lateral borders of the cartilage have been identified, an incision with a 15 blade is made at the junctions and a partial thickness cartilage graft is elevated. Ample cartilage will be derived from the graft for reconstruction. An attempt is made to avoid full resection and a discontinuous defect that hurts the patient more than when leaving at least a thin portion of continuous rib. However, when significant amounts of rib cartilage are required, it is best to obtain adequate volume even if it means taking some cartilage from 2 ribs to give the patient the best result possible (**Fig. 16**). Before final closure, hemostasis is

achieved and the wound irrigated. The donor site is then filled with saline and the anesthesia provider is asked to apply positive pressure to the lungs. An air leak will signify likely perforation and warrant further investigation and treatment. If no leak is detected, pneumothorax can be excluded. Avitene (Bard TM) or other collagen matrix can be placed into the harvest site before a layered closure to help with coagulation and dead space obliteration.

SUMMARY

Rhinoplasty for patients with cleft lip and palate is considered a very challenging nasal procedure. The goal is to restore symmetry, function, and nasal projection. A multifaceted and systematic approach is required to methodically reconstruct the nasal vault, primarily the nasal tip. Improving nasal projection is most often accomplished by septal extension grafting. Rib cartilage provides multiple advantages given its rigidity, volume, easy carveability, and resistance to postoperative

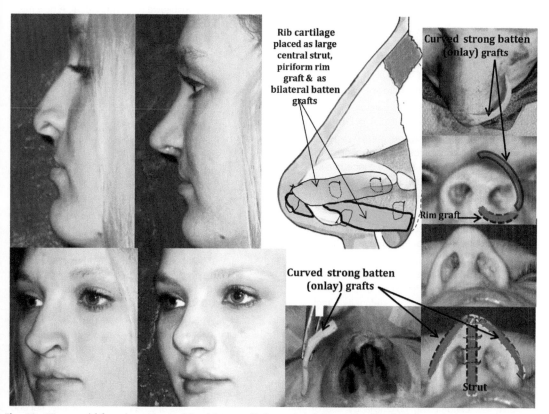

Fig. 16. 17-year-old female patient with a history of bilateral cleft lip and palate before and 4 months following rhinoplasty. Rib cartilage was used for a caudal extension graft, piriform rim grafts, and large batten grafts. The batten onlay grafts were extra indicated due to severe alar retraction in addition to the other common nasal issues involved with most cleft lip and palate patients. The bottom right diagram is total tip reconstruction using rib cartilage that is very useful for this challenging but rewarding set of patients.

scar contracture. Often overlooked is the deficiency in the premaxilla and piriform rim. The authors' experiences are that simultaneous grafting with cartilage or piriform rim implant will dramatically improve the aesthetics, especially when combined with other grafting techniques to augment and support the nasal tip. The patients tend to be extremely thrilled with results because their nose is often the only residual telltale sign of their cleft deformity.

REFERENCES

1. Sykes JM, Senders CW. Surgery of the cleft lip and nasal deformity. Oper Tech Otolaryngol Head Neck Surg 1990;1:219–24.

2. Sykes JM, Senders CW. Pathologic anatomy of cleft lip, palate and nasal deformity. In: Meyers AD, editor. Biological basis of facial plastic surgery. New York: Thieme; 1993. p. 57–71.

3. Sykes JM, Senders CW. Surgical treatment of the unilateral cleft nasal deformity at the time of lip repair. Facial Plast Surg Clin North Am 1995;3:69–77.

4. Blair VP. Nasal deformities associated with congenital cleft of the lip. JAMA 1925;84:185–7.

5. McComb HK, Coghlan BA. Primary repair of the unilateral cleft lip nose: completion of a longitudinal study. Cleft Palate Craniofac J 1996;33:23–31.

6. Huffman WC, Lierle DM. Studies on the pathologic anatomy of the unilateral hare-lip nose. Plast Reconstr Surg 1949;4:225–34.

7. Avery JK. The nasal capsule in cleft palate. Anat Anz 1962;109(Suppl):722.

8. Mulliken JB. Correction of the bilateral cleft lip nasal deformity: evolution of a surgical concept. Cleft Palate Craniofac J 1992;29(6):540–5.

9. Noordhoff MS. Bilateral cleft lip reconstruction. Plast Reconstr Surg 1986;78(1):45–54.

10. Stenstrom SJ. The alar cartilage and the nasal deformity in unilateral cleft lip. Plast Reconstr Surg 1966; 38:223–31.

11. Mulliken JB, Martinez-Perez D. The principle of rotation advancement for the repair of unilateral complete cleft lip and nasal deformity: technical variations and analysis of results. Plast Reconstr Surg 1999;104:1247–9.

12. Cronin TD. The bilateral cleft lip with bilateral cleft of the primary palate. In: Converse JM, editor. Reconstructive plastic surgery. Philadelphia: WB Saunders; 1964.

13. Cronin TD. Lengthening columella by use of skin from nasal floor and alae. Plast Reconstr Surg Transplant Bull 1958;21(6):417–26.

14. Garri JI, O'Leary K, Gabbay JS, et al. Improved nasal tip projection in the treatment of bilateral cleft nasal deformity. J Craniofac Surg 2005;16(5):834–9.

15. Bernstein L. Early submucous resection of nasal septal cartilage: a pilot study in canine pups. Arch Otolaryngol 1973;97:272–85.

16. Jablon JH, Sykes JM. Nasal airway problems in the cleft lip population. Facial Plast Surg Clin North AM 1999;7:391–403.

17. Crockett D, Bumstead R. Nasal airway, otologic and audiologic problems associated with cleft lip and palate. In: Bardack J, Morris HL, editors. Multidisciplinary management of cleft lip and palate. Philadelphia: WB Saunders; 1990.

18. Cho BC, Choi KY, Lee JH, et al. The correction of a secondary bilateral cleft lip nasal deformity using refined open rhinoplasty with reverse-U incision, V-Y plasty, and selective combination with composite grafting: long-term results. Arch Plast Surg 2012; 39(3):190–7.

19. Yan W, Zhao ZM, Yin NB, et al. A new modified forked flap and a reverse V shaped flap for secondary correction of bilateral cleft lip nasal deformities. Chin Med J (Engl) 2011;124(23):3993–6.

20. Rikimaru H, Kiyokawa K, Koga N, et al. A new modified forked flap with subcutaneous pedicles for adult cases of bilateral cleft lip nasal deformity: from normalization to aesthetic improvement. J Craniofac Surg 2008;19(5):1374–80.

21. Cheon YW, Park BY. Long-term evaluation of elongating columella using conchal composite graft in bilateral secondary cleft lip and nose deformity. Plast Reconstr Surg 2010;126(2):543–53.

22. Jackson IT, Yavuzer R, Kelly C, et al. The central lip flap and nasal mucosal rotation advancement: important aspects of composite correction of the bilateral cleft lip nose deformity. J Craniofac Surg 2005;16(2):255–61.

23. Wolfe SA. A pastiche for the cleft lip nose. Plast Reconstr Surg 2004;114(1):1–9.

24. Pitak-Arnnop P, Hemprich A, Dhanuthai K, et al. Panel and patient perceptions of nasal aesthetics after secondary cleft rhinoplasty with versus without columellar grafting. J Craniomaxillofac Surg 2011; 39(5):319–25.

25. Chaithanyaa N, Rai KK, Shivakumar HR, et al. Evaluation of the outcome of secondary rhinoplasty in cleft lip and palate patients. J Plast Reconstr Aesthet Surg 2011;64(1):27–33.

26. Huempfner-Hierl H, Hemprich A, Hierl T. Results of a prospective anthropometric and functional study about aesthetics and nasal respiration after secondary rhinoplasty in cleft lip and palate patients. J Craniofac Surg 2009;20(suppl 2):1863–75.

Cleft and Craniofacial Mission Care
Management of Facial Clefts: International Missions

Jeffrey J. Moses, DDS[a], Whitney J. Rochelle, DDS[b],*

KEYWORDS

- Cleft and craniofacial missions • Mission centers • Mission grants • Cleft and craniofacial teams
- International missions

KEY POINTS

- The best mission goal for teams working for facial cleft deformities is one of eventual establishment of a longitudinal treatment center.
- Considerations of site safety, regulations and permissions for operating foreign professionals, creating contacts with community organizations for support, patient screening, and quality and quantity of clean working facilities lay the groundwork for preparation before a site visit.
- Appropriate equipment is vital to the trip's success, such as power source, backup generators, instrument sterilization, need for portable water purifiers, and transportation arrangements for remote patients.
- Keeping the longitudinal treatment mission in mind, an organized method of establishing staged surgical care and follow-up visits for several years is crucial; the regularity of these schedules allows for adequate wound maturation between visits as well as facilitating the consistency of staged surgical care ongoing in a sequential fashion.

> The perfume of sandalwood,
> Rosebay or jasmine
> Cannot travel against the wind.
> But the fragrance of virtue
> Travels even against the wind,
> As far as the ends of the world.
> —Dhammapada

AMBASSADORIAL SERVICE

With all international missions, one must ask what exactly the "mission" is. What is hoped to be accomplished? Is it a personal goal of the visitor, or is it a personal goal for the host? I have found that the best mission goal for teams working for facial cleft deformities is one of eventual establishment of a longitudinal treatment center (**Fig. 1**), which includes all possible phases of care through a standard team approach for management. How this is accomplished is not important. I use the word mission in the same way as a military operative word is used, that is, a "project" so as not to confuse any religion's affiliation or context. Whatever one's personal convictions are will be passively demonstrated regardless of the pragmatic and sectarian nature of the goal of patient care.

PREPLANNING AND CONTACTS

When I am approached to help a foreign community with a mission startup, I always ask what exactly they perceive their needs are. Whether it is education, equipment, scholarships, our

[a] Smiles International Foundation (SIF), Oklahoma City, Oklahoma, USA; [b] Department of Oral and Maxillofacial Surgery, University of Oklahoma Health Sciences Center, Oklahoma City, OK, USA
* Corresponding author.
E-mail address: wjrochelle@gmail.com

Oral Maxillofacial Surg Clin N Am 28 (2016) 203–220
http://dx.doi.org/10.1016/j.coms.2016.01.001

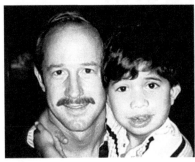
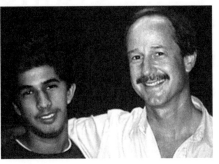

Fig. 1. This mission clinic child was operated for hemi-facial microsomia at age 4 and is shown at age 22 with Dr Moses at both ends of his treatment. Longitudinal care allows careful staged surgery and excellent follow-up.

operating either for them or side by side, and whatever that turns out to be, that is exactly what I arrange to provide and deliver to them. This process may have to be repeated several times, even at the same site, eventually filling up their "reservoir of needs" before the site is so completely "full" that they are brimming over, and it is then that they ask what else *they* can do to improve. They are then in a position that is ready to fulfill the original task and goal of the "mission." That is, to provide the children afflicted with facial cleft deformities sequential, longitudinal excellence of care and management appropriate to each deformity, which is performed at the proper time of growth and development. All this is done in order to achieve optimal results for the successful entry of that patient with optimal facial form and function into Society's membership.

This viewpoint is truly capitalistic because I feel when one is figuratively "full" and able to take care of all personal, professional, and familial needs, they then become more inclined to spiritually tithe or share a portion of their abundance in order to gain the joy that comes with giving and caring for those less fortunate.

This viewpoint has worked time and time again, and through the marriage of these clinics to international academic institutions as well as international service organizations, this process can be easily accomplished yielding a sustainable mission site, which has the very fabric of its community woven throughout thus ensuring its success.

The purpose of this article is to provide the reader with a concise outline of philosophic and practical knowledge for which to accomplish this goal of a sustainable and longitudinally oriented facial-cleft mission treatment center. The importance of longitudinal care cannot be overemphasized and is the foundation of an ethical and successful center for care. As a Foundation, we have had many opportunities to treat patients sequentially from stage to stage, participating in their marriages, sponsoring educations, and generally participating in expanded roles rarely available to our cross-sectional practices stateside. One such patient was portrayed by the famous Latino muralist, Mario Torrero, known for murals featured at the Vatican, who painted a work entitled, "Miraculous Metamorphosis" (**Fig. 2**), which was presented to the First Lady of Costa Rica, Gloria Bejarano (**Fig. 3**) and hangs in the Children's Museum in San Jose, Costa Rica, illustrating the stages of correction of the first patient of our mission work many years ago, which established the Costa Rica project, Smiles of Costa Rica (**Figs. 4 and 5**).

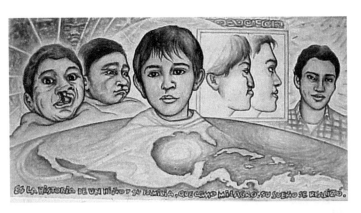

Fig. 2. The artistry entitled "Miraculous Metamorphosis," produced by famous Latino activist-artist, Mario Torrero, illustrating some of the stages of surgical care for the completion of a patient from Costa Rica. This art piece was presented to Costa Rica's First Lady, Gloria Bejarano, and currently resides at the Children's Museum located in San Jose, Costa Rica as a reminder of the successful establishing of the first Craniofacial Center in Central America at the Hospital de Ninos.

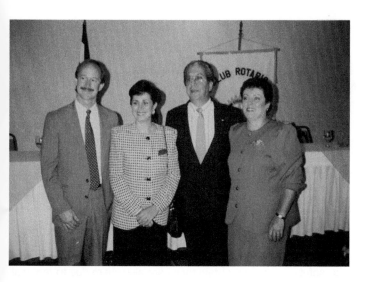

Fig. 3. The First Lady of Costa Rica, Gloria Bejarano de Calderon, second from left, Dr Moses, first left, and Rotarians Rodrigo and Lucia Sauma of the Club Rotario Rohrmoser, Costa Rica.

ADVANCE PLANNING AND CONTACT

I must acknowledge that I have learned that a team site is more easily developed and accomplished by strolling through, or even sometimes being pulled through, an open door, rather than by deciding on a locale and then pushing on that door in order to achieve it. All one has to do is to open space in their own calendar, open their heart and mind to a mission service, and the universe will conspire to fill that opening; you can trust me!

Once that opportunity presents itself to you, it is important to set your foundation in place to grow and form your mission site in a legitimate fashion. No matter the form of the invitation or opportunity request, I recommend always following the steps outlined in this article completely in order to be more certain of your long-term success. It is only fair for those children and families involved who have had their treatments initiated, so that they will not be "left hanging" with only partial treatments should the team fall apart later. The steps are as follows:

- Site appropriateness regarding team safety and security
- Licensure and governmental regulations
- Local clinician care and current facilities
- Community service organizations

From the comfort of your desk, you will want to research the governmental travel watch, such as

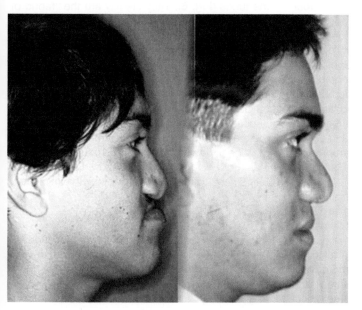

Fig. 4. Profile images of finished staged surgical case that was the case study for the artwork, "Miraculous Metapmorphosis," by Mario Torrero. His case was referred for treatment in the United States with Dr Moses, but instead was used as a catalyst to open the Craniofacial Unit at the Hospital de Ninos, Costa Rica, CR.

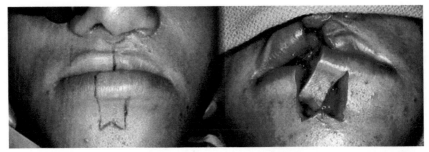

Fig. 5. These combined photographs illustrate just one of the many stages for the full facial reconstruction of cleft and craniofacial deformities. Abbe flap design and incision carried out on the patient portrayed in "Miraculous Metamorphosis" artwork shown in Fig. 2.

http://travel.state.gov/content/passports/english/alertswarnings.html, in order to ensure the site's appropriateness regarding your team's safety and security.

Contacts made to the proposed country's official state consulate or embassy can lead you to their regulations regarding foreign-trained professionals working and operating their profession within their country. They may refer you to that location's regional director of public assistance for the poor, who may have a more direct influence and can facilitate your permission to work with them (for example, in Mexico, this is the "DIF" or DESARROLO INTEGRAL DE LA FAMILIA; http://sn.dif.gob.mx/).

In addition, through contact to the president of the local active community organization, such as the Rotary Club, Lions, Kiwanis, and so on, you can find out about and contact local club members or their friends who happen to be physicians and dentists within that community. They may be willing to actually operate together with your team or provide preoperative and postoperative support for the patients. They can provide a valuable insight into the quality and availability of working facilities and hospital, knowledge of clean water and sanitation conditions, and equipment needs. Through their providing photographs of potentially available operating rooms and facilities, your nursing and anesthesia team members can get a general idea of facility equipment and conditions ahead of time in order to help them prepare for the eventual initial screening clinic and first site-visit.

Importantly, the community service organization can also act as a safety-catch to screen all potential patients and families so as to prevent damaging financial interferences with the area's private practice sector by accidently operating on a relatively wealthy customer who moves to the head of your screening line by societal dominance and who ordinarily would have been treated by their local private practitioners. This does not mean that you do not accept financially stable patients who cannot obtain their care elsewhere due to regional lack of that medical or dental specialty, nor those who are brought by their clinicians to work side by side for ambassadorial professional knowledge exchanges (*still, all treatments are performed free-of-charge by all parties in these cases*). Your team does not want to be known for operating on a case that had been scheduled only the following week by a local surgeon without his knowledge or approval, thereby risking being ostracized both professionally and governmentally.

Those community organizations, such as Rotary, many times provide necessary "boots-on-the-ground" assistance with transportation, customs negotiations at port of entry, lodging, and meals and can provide matching monetary grants for equipment needs of the project (if approached correctly), sometimes even hosting local fundraisers in order to supply their portion of the funds (**Fig. 6**). They literally are the "fabric of the community," participating as the business leaders of the community who apply much more weight of importance for continuity of support than many of the other usual vehicles used for surgical missions that I have seen in the past, which were supported through churches, military, school officials, and so on. This finding seems to be because this particular type of "fabric" outlasts regime changes within the government, churches, and local power infighting and has no religious bias. Following a phrase of action, *Service Above Self* seems to do the trick for everyone involved.

TEAM SITE VISIT AND TEST CASES

After a firmly established contact and location for the potential mission clinic is researched and verified to be permitted and welcomed, plans should be made for a physical site inspection visit, which may or may not involve being prepared for a

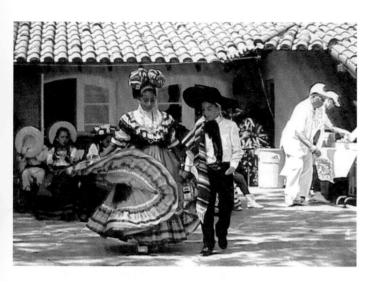

Fig. 6. Traditional Mexican folkloric dancers performing at one of the first fund-raiser dinner picnics hosted by Rotary for the development of funds for the Rotary Matching Grant, which purchased original equipment for the Thousand Smiles Cleft Center project in Ensenada, Baja California, Mexico.

performance of a test surgery or 2. In addition, a patient record-charting system is established, which can later be digitalized by your core team for off-site access, leaving the original paper records with the host facility. During screening, photographic records are taken after the parents or legal guardians have signed a treatment permission and photographic documentation and publication/social media usage release form, which is maintained and re-signed at each clinic (Appendix 1). On a separate clerical and legal note, it should also be a standard for your mission volunteers to sign a personal waiver of liability for any organizations connected with the program as well as ensuring any volunteers are either of legal age or have a legally appointed guardian present with them (Appendix 2).

The purpose of considering the possibility of a test case is to both motivate your site visit "core" professional team and flush out any potential needs of your support community, as well as the physical treatment facility itself so that future preparations will be made to be prepared for a full-team mission project.

With regard to your site visit's "core" team, it should minimally include the surgeon, anesthesiologist, operating room nurse, and recovery nurse. The recovery nurse can act as a circulating nurse during the first test case with the anesthesiologist managing the immediate postoperative recovery within the operating room together as a postanesthesia care unit until stabilized, depending on the level of care available at your chosen mission site. One of the nurses should be versed in postoperative cleft care nutrition and hygiene as well.

On the second visit, "core" members that can be added are the speech and language pathologists (**Fig. 7**) assisted by persons trained in nasopharyngoscopy (**Fig. 8**). General and orthodontic dentists (**Fig. 9**), audiologists (**Fig. 10**), and ear, nose, and throat specialists (**Fig. 11**), as well as clinical

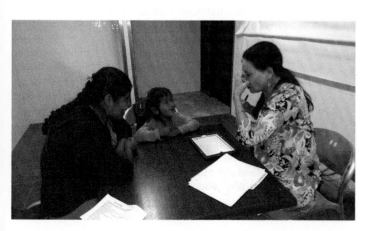

Fig. 7. One of our speech and language pathologists demonstrating where the nasal resonance sounds are felt to a young cleft patient and parent at the Smiles of Los Cabos mission project.

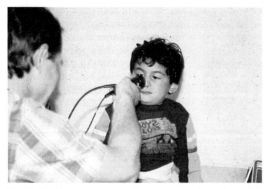

Fig. 8. Dr Moses preparing trust and conditioning with a patient before naso-pharyngoscopic examination.

psychologists or trained personnel experienced with the handling of self-esteem development, are added to the team for the establishment of longitudinal care and successful management (**Fig. 12**). On the occasion of establishing a craniofacial site, local neurosurgeons (**Fig. 13**), ophthalmologists, and genetic counselors have been used for complete team care.

Establishing a full-team approach to the management of the region's cleft and craniofacial population is the eventual goal of these project missions, and keeping that vision in the minds of both the volunteers and host clinicians is tantamount for success.

We have been blessed in setting up quarterly mission sites that have access for myringotomy tubes, ventilation, speech and language assessments and treatments, dental restorative care, orthodontic care followed by orthognathic surgery, and even dental implant restorative care into the grafted bone sites. All can be accomplished with proper growth of the team concept and added instrumentation within even a foreign mission

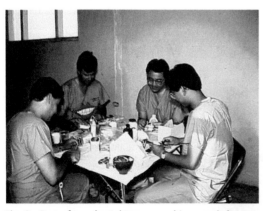

Fig. 9. One of our dental teams working on cleft management prosthetics and orthodontic palatal appliance construction at a cleft project in Mexico.

setting in time in some locations, even supplying mobile dental units through their community support organizations (**Fig. 14**).

It is always helpful to have an invitation extended to your mission site's local professionals to aid you with postoperative care, urging them to assist or somehow participate with this "first case" in order to assure firsthand knowledge of the case as well as to build team spirit and trust. Following a case completely throughout its treatment will let your team know what resources are already available and what needs should be enhanced for future expended clinics, whether via customs importation or via local purchases before the next planned clinic visit.

During the course of the site visit and before the test case, each member of the core team should make enquiry and inspect the various areas within their responsibilities (for example, auxiliary battery power and surge protectors, anesthesia machines, monitors, ventilation systems, intravenous fluid and administration set availability, as well as medications). Care must be given to ensure that the power plant for the facility has a backup electric generator, spare FULL oxygen tanks, and continuous water supply. If a functioning power backup generator is unavailable, there should be a plan to divert away from the common practice of use of the "all-in-one" monitor package popularly now used in anesthesia monitoring and revert to the independent critical patient-care monitors for noninvasive blood pressure system, O_2, CO_2, electrocardiogram, and so on, and any equipment necessary to safely complete the surgical case with each having their own independent battery backup pack installed and charged for when the "power-fail" occurrences come during critical moments. "Power-fail" occurrence has happened all too often on our trips, and preparation has saved the day more than once (**Fig. 15**).

Separate and secure storage rooms or a facility to store the mission team's special equipment and supplies between clinics are important to have built or provided. The specialty sterile supplies, extra sterilizer, anesthesia monitors, and other necessary equipment that were paid and provided by special grants specifically for the mission clinic will need to be stored and conserved in a dry, climate-controlled room with surge-protected electric power strips available (**Figs. 16** and **17**). You must know how much of this material remains on hand for the next clinic, and that it is functioning and available on return. You should be knowledgeable about standard restocking of the sterile supplies and disposables used and the amount that will be repurchased and shipped for the following trip. Of course, there are exceptions to this rule

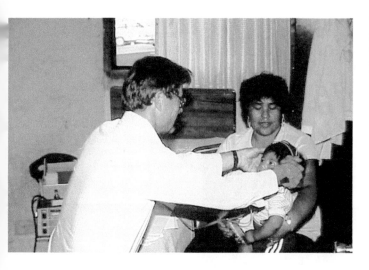

Fig. 10. One of our audiologists placing headphones on a child at one of our early cleft screening clinics in Ensenada, Baja California, Mexico.

for those equipment needs of the facility that your project has donated for their everyday use in improvement for the community, but, in general, because of equipment loss, breakage, nonmaintenance, and so on, it is wise to protect your mission clinic assets to ensure they are ready for you on arrival.

Battery backup units must be present within the monitors, and they need to be constantly attached to the surge-protected electric power strips during your absence so that they can cycle themselves and remain healthy. This facility should be built either within the hospital/clinic facility (if there is reasonable assurance of the clinic's continuing hospitality) or in a separate location of the supporting community service club's desire, assuming easy transportation of the storage material via their transportation assistance to whatever clinic facility will be designated for surgical care.

EXTRA CONSIDERATIONS
Operating Room Instrumentation Turnover Facilitation

Another consideration vital for rapid turnover and accomplishing the best use of donated service

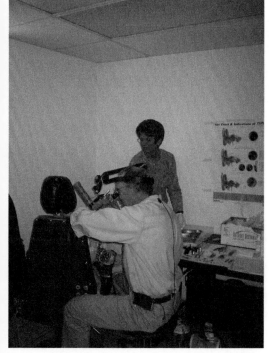

Fig. 11. Otolaryngologist, Dr Marc Lebovits, examines patient's auditory meatus to ensure previously placed myringotomy ventilation tubes are still functional.

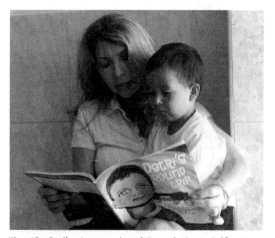

Fig. 12. Smiles International Foundation's Self-esteem and Patient Coordinator, Maribel V. Moses, reads to a troubled child from a relevant children's esteem development book, *Detri's Round Trip*.

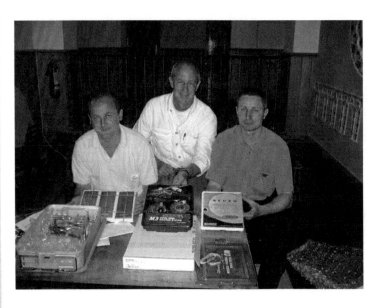

Fig. 13. Dr Moses (*center*) presents the grant donation for the specialized Neurosurgical Plating System to Smiles of Ukraine's Neurosurgeon, Dr Yuriy (*far right*), and Maxillofacial Surgeon, Dr Komok (*far left*), at the Smiles of Ukraine Craniofacial mission project.

time for mission care is how the instrumentation sterilization will be handled. Our experience has led us in many developing countries to quickly put a modern autoclave unit (EZ-10 E-Series automatic autoclave, Tuttnauer, U.S.A. Co) into the offered donation grant list early in the site development period. The result is a substantial increase in cases operated by twice the amount before the addition because the specialized and expensive instrumentation sets transported and carried by each team are in a limited supply, and through the judicious staggering of case scheduling for instrument set needs without duplication, a greater number of cases may be handled. The need for palatal retractors like the Dingman is ever present, and cases of pharyngeal flap, palatoplasty, fistula closures, and alveolar bone grafting all need to be interposed with cheiloplasty, rhinoplasty, external facial procedures, otoplasty, and so on, which do not require the Dingman and thus gives time for sterilization turnover. Having a reliable and modern automatic sterilizer in place will be a mission team enhancer and is easy to raise money for by the supporting organizations when the purpose is explained in such a manner (**Fig. 18**).

Water Health

In some countries or locations, a serious condition of contaminated water exists with not only the endemic risks for population dysentery and

Fig. 14. One of the surgical teams working at Thousand Smiles mission project early in project development standing next to a fully equipped dental treatment trailer donated by the Rotary Club for the project's use in the parking lot next to the surgical hospital. From left to right in the back row, Dr Jeff Moses, Dr Don Spengler, Dr Farrel Levasseur, Dr Tetsuji Tamashiro, Dr Kevin Smith, are identified and shown with numerous unidentified Rotaract and student volunteers.

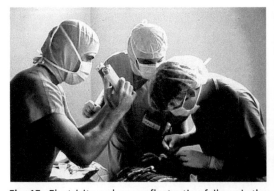

Fig. 15. Electricity and power fluctuation failures in the mission project field are frequent and point out the need for backup battery power systems on the anesthesia monitors as well as the need to have auxiliary battery flashlights available in the operating room.

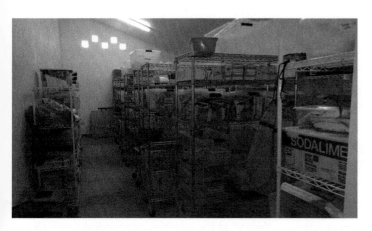

Fig. 16. A lockable storage room is crucial to having the specialized sterile supplies kept organized and inventoried as well as to keeping operating room equipment charged and ready for your ongoing scheduled mission project visits. This room was constructed by the Rotary Club of Tecate at their remote primary treatment clinic where we convert the unit triennially into a fully functioning operating and recovery treatment unit.

water-borne disease but also hospital water contamination with the postoperative risk of infections and possibility of resulting case failures. Usually the site visit can catch the risk factor, and plans for corrections via portable water purification systems (Custom Modular System: Water Mission International, North Charleston, SC) can be made before a full onset of mission clinic activities. However, there was one situation encountered where our site was very remote in the deltas of the Godavari River in Andhra Pradesh, Southeastern India, in which the village's well, orphanage, school residency, and hospital all drew water from a contaminated canal source, which served multiple purposes.

Swimming water buffalo, human waste runoff, clothing washing, dish washing, as well as human bathing were all done simultaneously with drinking and brushing of teeth from the same source! (**Fig. 19**). Needless to say, our water sampling tested positive for dangerous levels of various pathogens, including *Escherichia coli*, and we were forced to obtain water engineering in order to construct, ship, and install a water purification system (Custom Modular System: Water Mission International, North Charleston, SC) (**Fig. 20**). We

designed this to be sufficient for at least 6000 people and durable enough to last more than a 10-year lifespan requiring no expensive removable cartridges but rather scheduled backwashing, only the addition of an occasional swimming pool chlorine tablet and monthly water sample testing. Maintenance was taught to the hospital manager along with water sanitation courses at the school for the students and teachers alike (**Fig. 21**). This clean water unit supplied not only the hospital but also the orphanage school and dormitory serving more than 450 children and the local village as well of more than 4000 persons (see **Fig. 20**). It was a little tough to raise this up to the fourth floor of the tower near the tanks due to the absence of heavy equipment in this remote region, but it was made possible by old-fashioned hoist-and-tree-pole slide techniques (**Fig. 22**).

PATIENT AND CLINIC LOGISTICS

The possibility exists in some site visits to discover that the clinic provided is at a location that has the local support organizations, community support doctors, as well as accommodation and travel access, but does not have as many

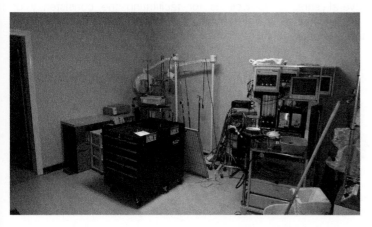

Fig. 17. Equipment stored in a dry, climate-controlled room with surge-protected electric power strips available.

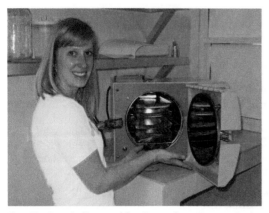

Fig. 18. One indispensable piece of equipment is the Automatic Autoclave Sterilizer purchased for your mission clinic in a size large enough to handle cranio-maxillofacial instrument sets and which can be set and operated by relatively inexperienced volunteer help so as to run constantly and assist in rapid instrument turnover, greatly enhancing the potential number of surgical cases handled each clinic. Care is to be given to use distilled water only and to review manufacturer's recommended usage with the team ahead of the busy operating day.

patients living nearby as those living rurally or many kilometers away. In these cases, making use of the community support resources, such as orphanages, Rotary or Lions or Kiwanis clubs, and possibly the governmental public family assistance organizations, which exist for that country (in Mexico, this is the DIF, which is present for every community; **Fig. 23**) and having access to vans or school buses, arrangements may be made for successful transportation for those families and patients to the regularly scheduled clinics and follow-up appointments for these groups on a scheduled basis.

On this note, it is imperative to point out that your team mission clinics must be scheduled in a fashion that everyone involved knows exactly your return clinic dates for the next several years.

This schedule will help your team volunteers, your host support team and hospital members,

patients and their families, and the community-at-large who are representing your future patient referrals to mark their calendars and reduce the potential for missed important follow-up surgeries and treatment care, giving you a longitudinal treatment line for your cases. In fact, many patients and their parents see these screening and treatment clinics as a chance to share experiences and to reconnect with others who share the challenges of living with facial differences. Some children have been on the same schedule for surgery as infants and matured over the years with their staged procedures at the same clinic look forward to seeing their surrogate "family" at the activities surrounding these clinics (**Fig. 24**).

I suggest never canceling a clinic, but if necessary, at least send an emissary to register the new patients, take follow-up photos of the old patients, and hold the door open until any issues are resolved. Too many mission sites have failed because of a loss of confidence of regularity and reliability.

I find that the most logical and consistent way to do this is by selecting your screening day and to call that day the repeating date. These clinics are usually held 2 to 4 times per year at the minimum so that consistent surgical timing can be given for wound healing between surgeries. For everyone's memory, it becomes useful to designate something like the "FIRST FRIDAY of each of the months of February, May, August, and November" for our quarterly weekend clinics such as the one I helped set up in Ensenada, Mexico held every 3 months. Or, as in the case of the clinic I helped set up in Cabo San Lucas, Mexico, working semiannually, which is known by all to begin on the FOURTH MONDAY of the months of April and October, giving 6 months between visits for this week-long surgical mission. The regularity of these schedules allows for adequate wound maturation between visits as well as for facilitating the consistency of staged surgical care ongoing in a sequential fashion.

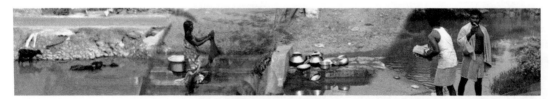

Fig. 19. This composite photo shows water buffalo swimming, women washing clothes and dishes, as well as men bathing and brushing their teeth in the same canals used for ingestion purposes at the orphanage kitchen, hospital, and school. All of this common usage adds up to filthy water sanitation and the presence of *E coli* in the drinking and cooking water both in the villages and at the hospital and kitchen at the orphanage clinic for Smiles of India.

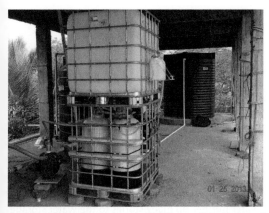

Fig. 20. A portable water purification unit is displayed here showing a compartmentalized unit, which is easy to install, requires only backwashing and no cartridges, exceeds US Environmental Clean Water Standards, and produces enough clean water for 6000 persons for over a 10-year lifespan (W.M.I. Portable Water Purification Unit).

Obviously, depending on whether each member of your team attends every clinic or only 1 or 2 throughout the year, this schedule can keep everyone's enthusiasm fresh and avoid "volunteer burnout." The avoidance of this is important to allow the eventual expansion of your program as it grows in size, being able to still give the necessary consistent care to your patients and families who, along with their friends, will spread the word that *you will always be there on those dates without fail thus far*.

Usually, if at all possible, it is helpful to schedule several days of surgery to allow for scheduling difficulties as well as missed

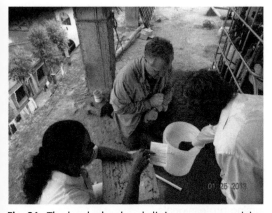

Fig. 21. The local school and clinic manager receiving instruction on weekly water testing and administration of backwashing procedures as well as the addition of chorine pool tablet as necessary from results of chlorine testing.

preoperative instructions allowing for alternate case fill-ins without condemning the conflicted case to a nonoperative status. These patients place a lot of hope on the surgery and travel a long distance at no small effort many times, and extra effort should be taken by the support volunteers in the town to put them up at a local orphanage or make arrangements for controlling their preoperative and postoperative environment as much as possible. However, on those "weekend" mission clinics spanning Friday to Sunday, I have found it advantageous to arrive Thursday evening and screen the first half of the day on the Friday, all the while looking for a couple of shorter revision cases that have yet to eat and are NPO (nothing by mouth). Then, isolate those select patients and bring them over for afternoon surgery. While the hospital team is cleaning the operating rooms and the recovery room and setting up the equipment, we continue the screening, preoperative evaluations, and follow-ups until they are finished, and the afternoon surgical cases are ready for induction.

Then, with a couple of minimally complex afternoon cases done, the wrinkles of any operating room delay-potentials are minimized, and all systems are made with a safe "go-ahead," ensuring a smooth and early start the next morning for the long and fruitful mission surgical treatment day. On the main operating room day, all operating rooms are therefore already set up, tested, and running well. The nurses and anesthesiologists can all get a good night's sleep, knowing the situation is well in hand for the next day, with having the final surgical scheduled cases arranged for morning admission planned with the necessary instrumentation presterilized and the cases reviewed that evening at the team's presurgical rounds and academic presentation.

Usually, in order to keep the professional team from burning out and happily returning each clinic, 5 to 6 cases are scheduled for each operating room available daily depending on complexity. I find that running 2 rooms as a minimum enhances the flow of the day due to staggered starting times and equipment overlap.

The team case review for the following day's surgeries can be done either before or after the team's continuing medical education (CME) lectures, which are brought to each mission in order to both enhance the team's appreciation of the management of the patient's facial cleft-care and to provide a platform for the International Ambassadorial cross-cultural exchanges of technique advancements as the mission site project grows.

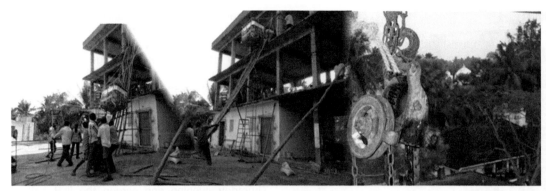

Fig. 22. Because there are no industrial cranes present in this remote village in India, old-fashioned ingenuity through the use of cut tree-poles was used to lift the 1-ton water purifier up many stories to the water storage tanks previously placed there for gravity distribution. Because of the size of the pump, the unit needed to be placed on the same story in this isolated instance. Inch by inch, with the assistance of many school workers and much prayer, the unit was slid up the poles by the use of the auto-engine hoist ratchet. Finally, the unit is received with success.

ACADEMIC AND AMBASSADORIAL EXCHANGE

It is helpful to have a US accreditation-certified continuing education provider available for your program because this gives all professionals valuable certificate verification of the course objectives and subject studies, which can enhance their curriculum vitae as well as serve for biennial license renewal requirements. Professional volunteers have limited free time in order to advance their CME requirements, vacation with their loved ones, and serve for charitable missions. The more you can accommodate these issues together, the more you will be assured reliable return of your carefully selected and experienced mission team providers. Not only do we provide CME and professional lectures (**Fig. 25**) but we also allow the members to bring their children at convenient times of their summer schedules to give their families first-hand interaction with volunteerism, starting them off with the preparation of food for the families of the patients and even allowing them to assist in the management of the children waiting for their surgical screenings. Some of these volunteer children have gone on for training and returned over the years as professional volunteers (**Fig. 26**).

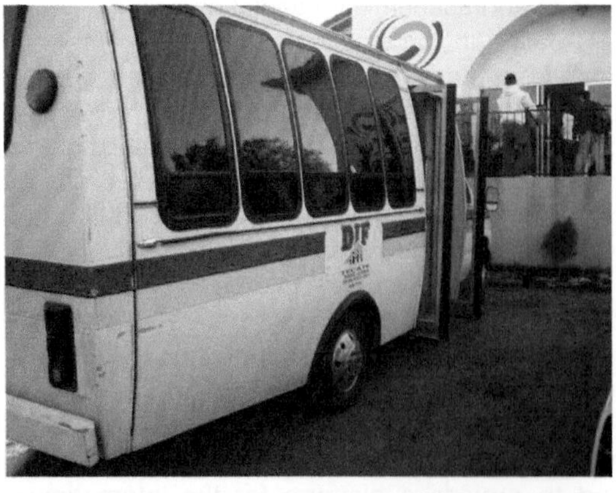

Sometimes the CME courses are presented either before or after the actual surgical days with invitations given to all of the local professional community with the assistance of the local Rotary or other service clubs who will host the auditorium. They may even elect to charge a nominal fee for the symposium lectures in order to gather funds for helping them offset their expenses in helping the programs for the children and their mission expenses. We have found this to be a mutually beneficial situation, which also serves to enhance the education of the local professional community on the patient care given and how they may continue that care throughout the year between clinics.

UNIVERSITY ACADEMIC AFFILIATIONS AND SUSTAINABILITY

We have found great stability for long-term success and sustainability to be provided by focusing responsibility for eventual "adoption" of your project mission site by a US-based academic institution, which has access to cleft/craniomaxillofacial surgeons, anesthesiologists, and dentistry and nursing professionals.

In addition to providing ongoing ambassadorial care for the children with modern and updated procedures and equipment, the host clinicians are able to share in international education

Fig. 23. Patient transportation vans like this one are often supplied for our patients by the community or governmental family assistance programs such as DIF in Mexico.

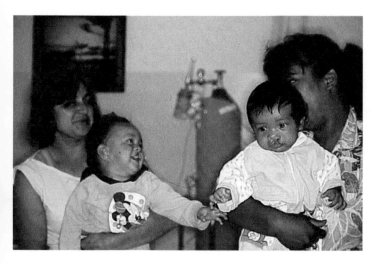

Fig. 24. Many children as well as their parents gain friendships over time and benefit from the longitudinal clinics occurring at the same dates several times per year to catch up on what might be expected later or to help the children gain friends. These friends may have a deep insight as to the social and developmental issues they face daily and can relate intimately. These clinics are sometimes the only chance for the children to see others who share their same facial differences, making them special friends.

exchanges and ongoing updates with sharing professional education opportunities. An example of this is the Ensenada, Mexico Thousand Smiles clinic we set up in 1985, which was groomed for adoption by the University of California at Los Angeles Oral and Maxillofacial Surgery Department. It has now entered its 31st year of quarterly operations; the Smiles of Los Cabos site in Southern Baja California, Mexico, adopted by the University of Michigan team, operates biennially. Each time a project mission site is developed, not only is thought and planning given to the eventual provision of leading specialty experts for a "full-team approach" for cleft care but also careful consideration is given to the exchange and invitation for academic leadership for sustainability and assurance of excellence of modern care.

In addition, the host site clinicians should be invited and sponsored to membership with the American Cleft Palate/Craniofacial Association (ACPA); we try to do this early in the process so we can instill in them an early vision of adherence to the Parameters for Evaluation and Treatment of Patients with Cleft Lip/Palate or other Craniofacial Anomalies (ref. revised edition November 2009: ACPA Parameters of Team Care, http://www.acpa-cpf.org/uploads/site/Parameters_Rev_2009.pdf).

We have examples of foreign members of our teams not only joining actively and attending these annual conferences but also availing themselves of visiting scholarship positions and taking the various techniques home, where their volume of cases greatly exceeded their US counterpart center mentors. Through their sharing of their professional experiences later, they have thus added valuable insights and statistical data to the international databases, reporting on evidence-based outcomes.

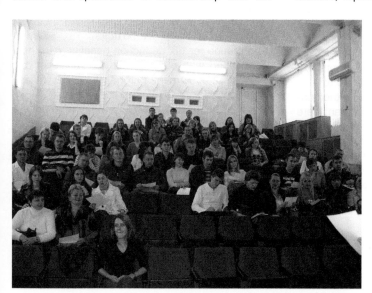

Fig. 25. A professional CME Symposium hosted by the Smiles International Foundation for the Mechnikov Medical Center professionals in Dnepropetrovck, Ukraine using the lecture from our visiting professors during their Craniofacial Cleft Surgical Mission Project, Smiles of Ukraine.

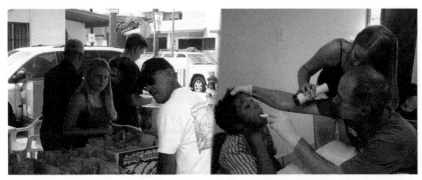

Fig. 26. This young woman is helping the volunteer Rotary group prepare lunches for the families and children obtaining professional treatments and screening during a mission clinic in Mexico. She also is shown helping hold a flashlight during an intraoral examination later that same day. Some of the families of volunteers have had their children become inspired with the charitable efforts and pursue medical/nursing careers themselves, and, due to the length of time of our clinics (more than 30 years thus far), have returned themselves to participate in their professional roles.

(An example of this is Dr Gabriela Saenz and the naso-alveolar-molding cases done at the Hospital de Ninos, San Jose, Costa Rica, with more than 1000 cases done in last several years in preparation for their cleft lip/nose procedures after her travels to the United States, arranged by the recipient of a Smiles International Foundation education grant for team experience resulting in the Center for Craniofacial Management at Hospital de Ninos, San Jose-Costa Rica; **Fig. 27**).

TEAM REPLACEMENT AND REGENERATION

"Succession for Children and Family's Treatment Continuity"

Sustainability with academic affiliation is only part of ensuring cases will be successfully followed with philosophic and technique continuity. In every project mission site, the team positions must be duplicated and regenerated constantly and consistently due to the process of "life happenstance" and the inevitability of changeover from these life events affecting the team members.

"A true leader is one who trains others to lead and provides his own replacement" (author unknown). Nowhere else, in my opinion, can there be a more sound philosophy applicable to provide this team preplacement and regeneration necessary for succession, which will ensure that the children and their families will have continuity of quality care in order for them to enter society as a fully functioning adult member.

FINANCIAL ALCHEMY
Matching Grants and Crowd-Sourcing

No project mission team article would be complete without mention of how to financially cover the

expenses. Although my personal philosophy has been to have a total "dog in the race" buy in by each professional volunteer and rely on the tremendous personal satisfaction reward that each of them gains from giving of their time, skills, finance for travel, and soul in the essence of service to others, I have become seasoned enough to understand that individual circumstances exist whereby this is not always possible for everyone at the volunteer level. If we wish to keep talented and caring individuals in the group for many years, some sponsorship must necessarily occur.

This sponsorship can be garnered in several different ways. Departmental outreach "charitable funding" given by the academic alumni, sponsorship for specialty residents and fellows from related equipment manufacturers, global and district financial grants from Rotary International and Districts who have been made aware of the international service project opportunities, and personal donations or tithes, which can ALL be placed into a Nonprofit 501(c)(3), Tax Exempt Organization for tax deduction benefits, can then be matched with other grants and multiplied by discounted equipment purchases, airline miles, and charitable travel agency contributions. All in all, it is not unusual to obtain a range of matched dollars from 4:1 up to 8:1 with the proper financial proposal preparations. This, with planning of what is needed, can provide your team and the host site with adequate equipment, which can stay in place for the ongoing surgeries (**Fig. 28**).

Again, by using the local project site's community support networks already present, such as Rotary or the other service nongovernmental organizations, many times they will donate meals and lodging, which lessens the financial load of the reliably returning volunteer professionals (for example, the Rotary Club of Tecate, Solmar

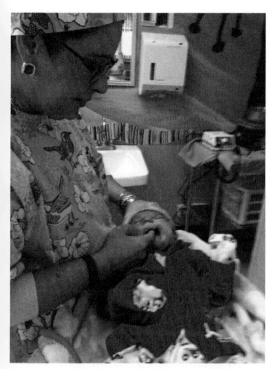

Fig. 27. Dr Gabriela Saenz is shown here preparing a naso-alveolar-molding appliance for a baby with cleft lip and palate at the Children Hospital in San Jose, Costa Rica. After the Pacific Clinical Research Foundation (Smiles International Foundation) presented her pediatric surgical colleague, Dr Roberto Herrera G, with a scholarship to attend the Parkland Memorial Hospital Craniofacial Unit, Dr Saenz joined him in Dallas, Texas and worked with Dr Andersen, later returning to Costa Rica to work with the technique in her cases at the newly formed Craniofacial Unit at the Hospital de Ninos. She has now more than 1000 cases treated with this approach and brings her experience with her to the meeting of the ACPA to compare results annually.

Foundation and Rotary Club of Los Cabos, and the DIF organization of Campeche with the Mayan Smiles missions all donate either all or part of the housing and meals for the visiting teams).

In fact, one good example of creative fundraising for local support is that done for many years by the Rotary Club of Rohrmoser, Costa Rica, who provided meals and hotels for our teams while developing the Craniofacial Center at the Children's Hospital in San Jose, serving all of the cleft population within the Central Americas who presented for care there regardless of country of origin. Because the team members brought with them professorial-level specialty-expertise from around the globe and had been invited speakers at numerous international conferences, the local Rotary asked our CME-accredited foundation to host symposia at each clinic to focus attention on the project as well as to give continuing education updates for the surrounding country's professionals and practitioners in the subjects of hypotensive anesthesia for craniofacial surgery, fiber-optic intubations, pediatric maxillofacial and cleft surgical techniques, dental implantology, and rehabilitation prosthetics for maxillofacial defects, among others. A small fee was gladly paid to the Rotary Club registering the participants and was considered by them to be a "donation" to the cause for the free surgical care by local practitioners, elevating their professional expertise as well as promoting knowledge of the care given with the project.

This and other community fund-raisers all supported the large entourage for the weeks of service several times annually in that country until they too began to be self-sufficient and sustainable with their own craniofacial center at the Children's Hospital.

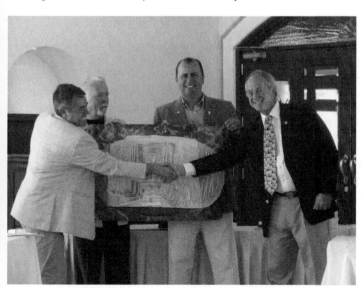

Fig. 28. Dr Moses (*far right*) is shown presenting a matching grant, which funded a large specialty equipment grant for the harvesting of bone for the craniofacial patients treated at the Smiles of Los Cabos mission project site. Also present in this photograph (*from right to left*) are Rotary Assistant Governor Cesar Rodriguez, Dr Mike McQuary, and Rotary President Oscar Nunez.

Of course, now we are also living in an age of crowd-sourcing, and one professional couple from Michigan showed me just how easy it is to crowd-fund a project, which was short a few thousand dollars for the purchase of sterile disposable supplies for one of their missions at the CaboSmiles site in just a matter of days enlisting a plea to help a child, *"Eat, Speak, and Smile."* This funding source should not be overlooked in this age of connectability to millions of souls via the Internet as a quick and readily available remedy for specific funds.

Regardless of your method or philosophy of funding, I do find that the more responsibility you place back onto each of the volunteers to either contribute or raise their own expense funding, the more dedicated and consistent a volunteer you will end up with. Give them a responsibility and ownership for their life of service, for we all strive for this eventually for fulfillment of our deeper life meaning. Responsibility builds resilience.

SUMMARY

I have discovered 3 truths in this journey of more than 41 years of charitable project mission care. One is to find and live the spirit of gratitude. Not only for all of the blessings found in our personal and professional lives but also for the opportunity to find an outlet for our inner need to serve in a meaningful fashion.

The second truth lesson is this: to live each day to the fullest and to do this with a true purpose of service to others. This lesson makes one stronger at the time when you feel those forces that are brought upon you and allow you to overcome them in order to be able to fulfill this chosen purpose, which is in need of your grateful service.

This brings us to the third truth. Be kind: to yourself and to others for any limitation or setback brought by one's own actions or externally. Everyone gets better through their struggles, and if you can only see this as a mechanism for growth, you can be forgiving and kind. With these 3 lessons in mind, it would be hard not to live a rich and rewarding life both personally and professionally.

Below are listed several service opportunity projects with their contacts. Although it is, by no means, complete or fully comprehensive, I hope it can give you some options to begin to serve as a surgeon who can share your specialized knowledge in the arena of cleft and craniofacial project mission care.

Definition of greatness: "Someone who looks back daily and says, 'I did something of worth,'" Eric Greiter, PhD, Rhode Scholar, Philanthropist, Naval Seal.

Volunteer Opportunity Contacts

Drawing Alegria
    Contact: Francisco Garzon, Executive Director Canada
    francisco@fgteam.ca
    905-275-9400
    Volunteer Link: http://drawingalegria.com/about-us/

Facing Futures Foundation
    Contact: Barry Steinberg, MD, PhD, DDS, Founder
    Volunteer Link: http://facingfutures.org/index.html

Free to Smile
    Contact: Byron Henry, DDS/Stacy Henry, Founders
    Volunteer link: http://www.freetosmile.org/

Mercy Ships
    Contact: Donald K. Stephens, Deyon Stephens, Founders
    Volunteer Link: http://www.mercyships.org/

Operation of Hope
    Contact: Jennifer More Trubenbach, President
    jtrubenbach@cox.net
    949-463-1795
    Volunteer Link: http://operationofhope.org/?utm_content=drjeffmoses%40yahoo.com&utm_source=VerticalResponse&utm_medium=Email&utm_term=http%3A%2F%2Fwww.operationofhope.org&utm_campaign=A%20fun%20Blessing%20update…%20Union%20Tribune%2C%20San%20Diegocontent

Sharing the Journey International
    Contact: David Cunning, DMD, Jacqueline J. Cunning, PA-C, Founders
    Volunteer link: http://stji.org/

Shares International
    Contact: Michelle Gross, Executive Director Florida
    Michelle.Gross@flhosp.org/
    Volunteer Link: https://www.floridahospital.com/shares/understanding-our-mission/cleft-lip-and-palate-program

Smiles International Foundation
    Contact: Jeffrey J. Moses, DDS, FAACS, Founder/President
    Volunteer Link: http://smilesinternationalfoundation.org/home0.aspx

Uplift Internationale
    Contact: Jaime Yrastorza, DMD, Founder
    Volunteer Link: http://www.upliftinternationale.org/about-us/uplift-international-board-of-directors/

APPENDIX 1

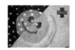

Patient Record/Photograph Use Consent Document

The surgery on_____(name of patient) is supported by the Smiles International Foundation (SIF) as an international children's charity working to eradicate the prevalence of cleft lips and cleft palates.

SIF maintain medical records on the patients undergoing surgery. These records include information such as: the names and addresses of patients and their parents, clinical diagnosis, other relevant medical health information, surgical procedures and results. The records also include pictures and videos.

SIF uses these records for reviews of surgical quality, education, evaluation, and public relations and marketing and promotional purposes as well as use in social media by the persons working during the clinic. The personal health information contained in the medical records will be maintained by SIF. Authorized persons, such as physicians, publishers, and promotions and marketing personnel as well as other medical personnel will have access to the records and the database and be able to use this for Smiles International Foundation purposes.

Additionally, SIF will keep your health information private and confidential by implementing security standards that limit access to the database to only authorized personnel as determined by SIF. SIF also will allow you to view the data contained in the medical record database and remove your name and health information from the database upon request.

I understand the information written above. I give my permission to send Smiles International Foundation a completed Medical Record Form for myself (if of the age of majority in proper jurisdiction) or my son or daughter from any other medical provider.

I give Smiles International Foundation to use this health information for quality assessment, education, evaluation and public relations purposes as well as for marketing, book and article publications. This permission includes use in the social media including Facebook, Twitter, Email, or other Internet Forums. I understand that this media may result in the information used to be accessible indefinitely, and may be unable to be erased or removed from the digital cloud.

_____   _____

Signature of Patient/Parent/Guardian (Circle)   Date

_____   _____

Signature of Witness   Date

APPENDIX 2

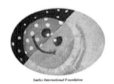

<u>Registration and Waiver of Liability</u>

Print Name of Participant: _____

Participant Address: _____

_____

Phone: _____ Cell: _____ Fax: _____

E-mail: _____

In case of Emergency Call or Contact:_____

Phone_____

I am aware of the risks associated with participation in a medical mission to _____ [name of country] which is supported by Smiles International Foundation for which I have volunteered. Accordingly, I, for myself, my heirs, representatives or assigns, hereby unconditionally release the fore-mentioned, its agents, representatives, employees and other volunteers from any liability whatsoever arising from such risks including, but not limited to death or personal injury by accident, sickness, disease, weather, terrorism, damage or theft which may be sustained by me as part of the medical mission to _____ [name of country] in which I will be participating. I know, understand and appreciate these risks and knowingly assume them.

Participant's Signature: _____

If Minor Participant's Parent/Guardian Signature _____

Date of Signature: _____

Using 501c3 Foundations in the Care of Cleft and Craniofacial Children

Kevin S. Smith, DDS[a,b,*], Byron T. Henry, DDS[c,d]

KEYWORDS

- Foundation • Mission • Overseas • Board of directors • Fundraising • Cleft lip and palate
- International

KEY POINTS

- Initiating a medical nonprofit foundation requires a great deal of thought, effort, and care.
- To begin and sustain a medical nonprofit, several aspects of the foundation need to be explored and put into action, all of them necessary for success.
- The board of directors, the very cornerstone of any nonprofit foundation, is crucial to the energy, everyday tasks, and decision-making to allow for true success.
- Growth, funding, and accountability are all aspects of a nonprofit that need attention, thought, and action.
- Starting a nonprofit, either locally or internationally, involves a very steep learning curve with many successes and failures along the way; yet creating a vehicle that only has the goal to help others without expecting anything in return is incredibly rewarding and fulfilling in life and will never be looked on with regret.

DOMESTIC FOUNDATION: A SMILE FOR A CHILD FOUNDATION, OKLAHOMA CITY

Initial Founding

A Smile for a Child Foundation was set up in 2003 after I experienced frustrations taking care of children who fell outside the Medicaid system and did not have the financial resources to take care of the cleft-required treatment for lip and palate. Specifically, the biggest need that they had was speech therapy, dentistry, and orthodontic care. The concept of a local foundation to help children with facial deformities sprang from frustration primarily with orthodontic care for children with cleft and craniofacial deformities. We had enlisted help from virtually every orthodontist in the state of Oklahoma, many of whom graciously treated many of the kids gratis. We thought that if we could raise funds for children who fall outside the Medicaid system to help with the costs of speech, dentistry, and orthodontics, we would establish a mechanism for treating all children within the state of Oklahoma. Everyone reading this article knows the heartstrings that are pulled for children with cleft and craniofacial deformities, and all of us have noticed advertisements by the large international charities, such as Smile Train and Operation Smile. We thought that if we could harness contributions within Oklahoma to help Oklahomans by using this same "heartstring-type" marketing, we could establish a system that would deliver care to all children in Oklahoma.

Initial thoughts on the founding of the charity revolved around whether to do it within the university setting or in a private community fund. Certainly

[a] JW Keys Cleft and Craniofacial Clinic, A Smile for a Child Foundation, University of Oklahoma, Oklahoma City, OK, USA; [b] MK Chapman Cleft and Craniofacial Clinic, University of Tulsa, Tulsa, OK, USA; [c] Free to Smile Foundation, University of Oklahoma, Columbus, OH, USA; [d] University of Oklahoma, Oklahoma City, Oklahoma, USA
* Corresponding author. MK Chapman Cleft and Craniofacial Clinic, University of Tulsa, Tulsa, OK.
E-mail address: Kevin-Smith@ouhsc.edu

Oral Maxillofacial Surg Clin N Am 28 (2016) 221–228
http://dx.doi.org/10.1016/j.coms.2016.01.002
1042-3699/16/$ – see front matter © 2016 Elsevier Inc. All rights reserved.

the advantages of doing this within the university setting include already established resources and marketing techniques to, it was hoped, push funds into this foundation. Disadvantages were evident immediately, in that the administration of the university foundation made it clear in no uncertain terms that certain donors could not be approached for contributions to our foundation and that they had been tagged for contributions to the university in general. This limitation of who was approachable and who was not pushed the establishment of the foundation within the private sector. Within most cities, there are conglomerate groups of charitable organizations that exist. In Oklahoma City, it is in the form of the Oklahoma City Community Foundation. The Oklahoma City Community Foundation houses hundreds of 501c3 foundations and is able to provide initial charitable status via an umbrella through their 501c3. A Smile for a Child Foundation was established within the Oklahoma City Community Foundation as essentially a fund managed by them. Any contributions were considered tax exempt due to the umbrella from the Oklahoma City Community Foundation.

Infrastructure

The infrastructure of setting up a foundation can perhaps be the most challenging aspect. Initially, bylaws and articles of operation need to be established. Establishing a functional board can be a challenge. It is absolutely necessary to get the right type of people on the board, people who are not afraid to ask for contributions and believe in the mission of your foundation. In addition, the board needs to be made up of people who can perform different tasks within the foundation. If you chose all health care providers, then you may be missing services of accounting, banking, and marketing.

For A Smile for a Child Foundation, the biggest hurdle was pushing through the 501c3 application. The process took several years, which may come as a surprise, but this was due to identified problems within the foundation itself. The identified problem was me. As medical director of the foundation, it was very difficult for me to delegate duties and powers to other board members. Once the realization of delegation of powers and duties took place, the foundation started clicking. Once delegation occurred, establishment of other infrastructure items like stationery, Web pages, electronic contribution methods, brochures, and a host of other items needed to properly run a foundation actually occurred.

The hiring of an Executive Secretary is paramount to success. One struggle for young foundations is seeing money raised that in your mind is supposed to go to treating children going to salaries. This false sense of money preservation must be overcome early because it is of the utmost importance to have someone looking at the work of the foundation on a daily basis. If you establish or help establish a foundation, make yourself a permanent member of the board but "let it go." You must establish a board that knows what the task is that needs done and then let them do it.

Fundraising

The most consistent form of fundraising has occurred in the form of small donors, usually stimulated by some association of a patient with a cleft or craniofacial disorder. With a simple brochure, contributions by small donors have done very well. Additional methods of fundraising include a local high school that has a fundraising week. The high school adopted A Smile for a Child Foundation for their fundraising efforts. An unbelievable $142,000 was raised by the Edmond Memorial High School in Edmond, Oklahoma.

Additional methods of fundraising include simple money boxes placed at participating health care offices with solicitation for matching money contributions made into the box. This money box routine should be used during the month of July, which is the cleft and craniofacial awareness month. The issue with money boxes is that many times they are neglected by the office staff of the participating office. If no one "owns" the cause, the money box will just sit unattended. Perhaps a better way to enlist dentists, physicians, and other professional offices is to secure a contribution from them based on the patients they see over a period of time. For instance, "My office will contribute $1 for every patient seen in July" or "I will give 1% of collections in the month of July." In this manner, we can simply place "Thank-you" signs in the office for their amazing contribution.

Many foundations hold a gala every year, but your board has to be very active and have organized and coordinated efforts into pulling that gala off. These coordinated efforts include soliciting materials for auctions, door prizes, venues, food, and entertainment. The list of fundraising opportunities is only limited by the imagination of your board.

Distribution of Funds

Recently, an evaluation of all funding expenditures for the foundation was conducted. Because of the volunteer nature of the board, the overhead expenditures of the foundation have been minimal.

Overhead expenditures have included infrastructure items, such as Web page, contribution boxes, literature, mailings, and lunches for board meetings.

Most funds raised are used by A Smile for a Child Foundation for the direct benefit of children with craniofacial disorders. More than 50% of the distributions have been for care of patients in the form of reimbursement to the orthodontists, dentists, speech pathologists, and audiologists that were taking care of these children. By far, most of the expenditures have been for orthodontics. One philosophy of the foundation includes making sure that everyone has "skin in the game." Orthodontists are asked to forward a treatment plan for the patient and provide some form of discount for the patient's care. The patient is then asked what amount of the financial obligation to the provider they can pay, and the foundation makes up the difference through direct payment to the provider. The philanthropy of the orthodontists has been incredible. Typically, they provide anywhere from 10% to 25% discounts off their treatment plan rate. The patient typically will make a payment plan for 50% owed, and the foundation ends up paying the remaining 50%.

Less than half of the expenditures from A Smile for a Child Foundation have gone to indirect patient care. The University of Oklahoma and the University of Tulsa have received the bulk of these grants. The grants are used for the purchase of special needs feeders. Each of the cleft clinics at the University of Oklahoma and the University of Tulsa uses funds to purchase special needs feeder, such as Haberman Special Needs Feeder (Medela, Inc, McHenry, IL), Pigeon cleft feeder (Phillips Respironics, Murrysville, PA), and Dr Brown's cleft bottles (Dr. Browns, St. Louis, Mo). The purchase of these bottles has a great effect on referral patterns to the cleft clinics because patients understand that they can get free bottles. There is an amazing thing that happens when you tell parents who are already stressed with a cleft child that they can get bottles for free. They have already done the research and found them online for $30 to $40. They realize the value of the Foundation and the cleft team immediately.

In addition, the professionals at the cleft clinics have purchased cleft-specific instrumentation to facilitate the diagnosis and treatment of cleft lip and palate patients.

Patients can apply for foundation money with an application available on our Web site. Evaluation of the application is needs-based and done by an independent social worker. In general, families with children with cleft and craniofacial disorders have significant expenditures related to these diseases, and so far, no one has been denied grants.

One thing of importance to note is that A Smile for a Child Foundation does not typically fund surgery. One reason is that I typically am the surgeon and a member of the board, so to avoid a definite conflict, surgery is not funded unless it is for another surgeon or dentist. The advantage we have in our state is that another foundation exists that funds area children's surgical needs. We write grants to this foundation on a regular basis.

Longevity of the Foundation

Foundations are only as good as their boards and their fundraising opportunities. One goal of A Smile for a Child Foundation is to place a percentage of funds raised each year into endowed funds. Within the Oklahoma City Community Foundation, there are specific foundations that will match funds placed into endowed funds, generally 2:1. Consequently, if $30,000 is placed into endowed funds, an additional $15,000 would be granted by this other foundation. The ultimate goal of our foundation is to establish large amounts of endowed funds so that our foundation can act on a longitudinal plan to affect the health of children with cleft and craniofacial deformities in the state of Oklahoma.

The board will play a major role in the longevity of the foundation. Board members who have lost interest in the foundation need to be replaced with new, enthusiastic members. Each time a board member has been replaced, A Smile for a Child Foundation has made new strides in achieving their goals. Paying for an executive director is paramount to moving forward. Even though this expense is significant for young foundations, it is important for someone to be paying attention to the foundation on a daily and weekly basis.

As said earlier, part of the problem with advancement of A Smile for a Child Foundation was me, and this is due to the fact that I was trying to run virtually all aspects of the foundation. With the appointment of an executive secretary who was paid for services, all aspects of running the foundation, from appropriate spending of monies for infrastructure to organizing the next fundraising event to providing care for patients, are kept on track.

One of the difficult tasks of foundations is to keep on track with the goals of the foundation, which is patient care versus just concentrating on fundraising. You must be diligent in identifying patients who need help, because this, in turn, will provide the foundation with higher visibility and long-term survivability.

INTERNATIONAL FOUNDATION: FREE TO SMILE FOUNDATION, COLUMBUS, OHIO
Initial Founding

It has been my privilege to both participate and lead surgical cleft missions for the past 15 years. Working in impoverished countries in more than 50 surgical missions has led to both professional and personal changes in my life, all of them being more rewarding than I would have ever expected. My first 8 years of surgical missions was accompanying various respected organizations that perform such work and learning the art of cleft surgery. It was exciting, educating, and stimulating all at the same time. This love of cleft children along with the intense changes in my life brought on by these missions hooked me and set me on a life quest to continue to help these children as long as my skills would permit me to do so. To both my surprise and my naive nature, I learned that there is so much more to these missions than the life-changing surgeries they provide. I realized that the surgeries all result from a tremendous amount of work and preparation that goes into making a mission come to fruition. They are possible because of the nonprofit foundations that make it all happen.

The scope of the missions I have joined ranges from an immense amount of coordination between host countries, fundraising, team recruitment, an overwhelming list of administrative duties, and a preparedness among so many key players on the team. A volunteer on the outside never would realize all these things. As I learned more and more throughout the years, I also became frustrated by so many aspects of mission work. Among them were egoism, unpreparedness, disorganization, improper facilities, dangerous anesthesia, and "rogue" missions that, quite frankly, compromised the surgeries and in some cases may have done more harm than good.

As I continued to accumulate enough knowledge and learn from those who have gone before me, I knew my ultimate goal was to create my own nonprofit organization and lead these missions. Admittedly, I was naive then and altruism was winning over the reality of the work that goal would involve, but I knew in both my mind and my heart that it was a goal I wanted to achieve. I was armed at that point in my cleft experience with enough skill and had raging motivation and confidence. I honestly had so much to learn though.

Fast-forwarding 7 years, I look back now and realize, as scary as it may have seemed, and as many mistakes as I surely have made, founding Free to Smile (FTS) was one of the best ideas I have ever followed through to fruition. There have been many bumps in the road, and no foundation ever succeeds by the work of one person but is instead the result of joint efforts by individuals, corporations, donors, and so much more. In the end, I realized that the true goal of any surgical cleft mission is to help the children who suffer so much from this congenital deformity. Such missions are only possible through nonprofit foundations that unite great humanitarians who donate talent, time, and money to change lives. I knew I had to be part of that bigger effort and began my own nonprofit foundation, FTS, in 2008. It has been in existence for 7 years and continues to grow, learn, and provide surgeries to children in need all over the world. To date, FTS has completed 35 surgical missions, performed more than 450 cleft surgeries, and changed the lives of not only patients but also volunteers. FTS continues to get better and more efficient each year. In this article, I share some of my experience and the knowledge I have gained over the years regarding what makes a cleft nonprofit successful from a surgical perspective as well as a business perspective.

Board of Directors

Nonprofits exist to accomplish social or service goals and always need ways to stay focused on their mission. In my experience, most nonprofits are launched on a wing and a prayer rather than a well-thought-out plan. It is often passion and motivation that start them rather than clear understanding of what is takes to make it grow and keep it focused and running successfully. It cannot be overstated how important a board is for a nonprofit's success. It is the very lifeblood and extension of the organization. Essentially, it acts as the "voice" in the community, and the world, if it is an international entity. When I first assembled our board, I was interested in people who knew my mission work and shared my passion. I approached people I had close relationships with, most of whom I knew for several years. The initial board included 5 people: 3 dentists, 1 attorney, and 1 teacher. Our board remained the same for the first 3 years. I would say we were all equally motivated and focused for about 2 years. Then came a period of stagnation for, I think, various reasons, including lack of diversity within the board and unclear goals. I do not think we really understood what a board is truly supposed to accomplish. As we grew, we realized that we want and need a board with a mix of skills ranging from financial, technical, entrepreneurial, legal, administrative, and social service. That said, I continue to believe that passion and commitment are just as important, if not more so, than specific skills. To find someone that serves as an extension of your mission in the community and the world is a rare thing and will undoubtedly bring success to your nonprofit. I have learned that sometimes those who look great on paper do not have the commitment and enthusiasm necessary to promote the cause.

FTS currently has 7 board members, including 3 of the original founding members. Members are volunteers and have never been compensated, with the exception of our executive director (and cofounder), who gets compensated a small salary. In the early formation of the board, we did not implement limited terms for members. As the years went by, I realized that this is a critical part of the board, with maybe the exception of the founder(s). Over time, board members can become weary of the cause; they lose focus and no longer advocate for the mission actively. The board is at its best with members who stay focused and remain involved and zealous.

Development of our board has been a true learning experience with many bumps in the road. We did not realize at the beginning that a nonprofit is ultimately a business and needs to run like a business. Every business needs a plan, and the responsibility and roles of the board members need to be clearly stated and outlined. We now have legal contracts and very clear outlines of what the roles of each board member are in the organization. I have found that clearly defined goals, which you may think would be intimidating to your selected members, actually allow them to stay focused and lead to much more success.

As each year passes, we become more organized, with clearer goals and new members leading the way for FTS. A widely diversified, highly motivated board of directors can lead to real success in accomplishing the mission of your foundation. A final lesson learned is that FTS's "worker bees" are equally, if not more, important than those with highly defined skills. It always takes an army to move mountains.

Fundraising

As stated above, I started FTS on a whim; I never looked at it as a business but rather a passion. In reality, a nonprofit is essentially no different in context than a for-profit entity: at the very least, it needs to flow as much money in as what goes out each year or it will never succeed. That is, those who need help will not receive it.

It was always a bit intimidating asking for money in the beginning from friends, relatives, and a host of others, but there are very few human beings who would not lend a hand to others who need help in life. All we have to do is ask. After year 3, I realized that a succinct, frank business plan and fundraising goals are absolutely essential to the success of a nonprofit. It took me a while to realize this, but successful nonprofits have a laid-out plan and review it often. FTS created this plan in year 4 and, looking back, it has been one of the key milestones in making us successful. For the first 3 years, we were "running on a shoestring." With the advent of a focused business and fundraising plans, we had the potential to focus and grow as a board. The plan changes annually, and we review it on a regular basis. We discuss our goals at every board meeting, 4 per year, but focus on them most closely at our annual meeting each year. At this meeting, we look at the year ahead and decide all of our fundraising goals, our mission goals, and our budget. The board of directors has many decisions to make at that meeting and oftentimes a follow-up meeting is required (**Figs. 1** and **2**).

With respect to fundraising, in the beginning, most of our funds came directly from charitable contributions from individuals. It took a solid 2 years of lecturing and presentations to turn FTS into a solid, well-known, and respected entity. I think with that respect and a bit of longevity came a new sense of confidence to ask for donations from individuals and corporations and apply for grants from various sources. Some of this came from greater awareness of what is available and some from growing confidence. We began to see a steadiness in our funding that allowed us to create some sense of a budget. Most of our donations into year 7 came from foundation grants, family foundations, corporate philanthropy, and growing charitable contributions from individuals. The main lesson in fundraising is that it is a wheel that needs continually spun. A nonprofit cannot rest and assume that because a donor made a

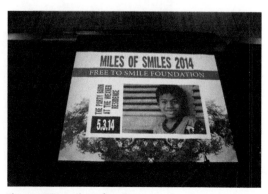

Fig. 1. FTS's miles of smiles annual gala presentation poster.

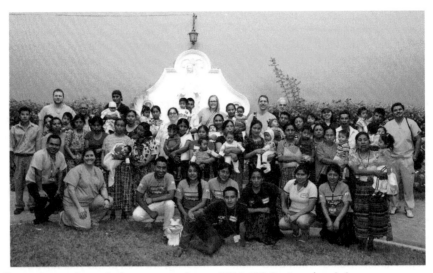

Fig. 2. Families gather at the end of surgery week on a 2014, FTS Guatemala mission.

contribution the prior year, he or she will donate again this year. Continual stimulation and proof that the mission is being achieved are essential to keep the donations flowing into the nonprofit. It takes continual effort and, in my experience, it takes at least 5 years to establish a solid donor base of grants, corporate efforts, and charitable contributions (**Fig. 3**).

Growth

Sooner or later, every nonprofit contemplates the risks and rewards of expanding beyond its original charter. The fact of the matter is that many, many more nonprofits fail than survive. It is estimated that more than 100,000 nonprofits nationwide fail every 2 years. This challenging time when you confront growth as an organization draws upon the board of directors to examine the benefits, drawbacks, and challenges of organizational growth and managing this growth in a way that maximizes the mission and its impact on the world. This aspect of FTS has been and continues to be a very difficult task for our board of directors. Positive growth occurs to meet an unmet demand. With so many charities in existence performing cleft lip and palate overseas on medical missions, how does FTS address a demand that is unmet? How do we measure quality, which can also be a symbol of growth? Growth for a nonprofit is usually assumed to mean an increase in financial income, but growth, in truth, can mean so many other things: quality, exposure to the public, increase in service offered. In this case, that is surgical care.

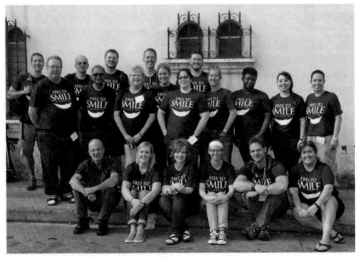

Fig. 3. Surgical team for FTS's 2014 Guatemala mission in Guatemala City.

I was brutally naive in the beginning. I assumed that organizational growth was automatic, and all I needed to do was to talk about it and it would grow. What I have learned is that growth will only result from a reasonably and closely managed process. This, too, falls on the board of directors: to determine the feasibility of this growth. To date, FTS still toils with the questions of where and how to grow. Do we add more programs or missions sites? Do we add to the amount of patients to each site that we can operate on? Do we spend more on marketing to grow? The questions and the possibilities are endless, and the reality is that it does not make sense for an organization to grow or expand in a way that sacrifices program quality or any mission, or jeopardizes the financial health of the organization.

The reality for FTS is that we accumulated more money than we ever thought we could, and we thought it was best to expand into different countries. What we learned was that when we grew too fast we began to overburden the administrative staff; we were not able to find enough mission volunteers in a timely manner, and we lost focus on our existing programs. Fortunately, as an organization, we were able to reboot and refocus and realized that slow, steady growth with quality is better; again, resorting to the very meticulous well-thought-out plan that always makes sense.

As a founder, I was trying to expand my skills, always being fearful that if I did not move in that direction, another cleft mission would take over. What I realized is that quality far outweighs how many surgeries your organization can perform over the year. On a great track presently, our plan is to continue to expand, but very slowly and with steady focus on quality. This plan shows your donors and corporations that you care about your work and the money they donate. Slow, steady, and quality growth always comes out victorious.

Accountability

Accountability is a buzzword in today's nonprofit world. Organizations continue to find themselves under the microscope of public scrutiny after so many publicized and scandalous events in recent years. Rightly so, I might add. There are no monitoring forces or governing bodies to oversee or streamline the operations of a nonprofit organization. These fears of the public about nonprofit organizations are justified. Who will ensure that money given is spent wisely? Who will guarantee desired outcomes? Are these nonprofits operating within tax exemption and fundraising laws?

This list of questions can go on forever, and they certainly were questions and facts that I had absolutely no idea about when I started FTS Foundation in 2008. What I have learned is that accountability is the backbone of any nonprofit organization. Without standards of accountability, we can and will lose the trust of the public. Loss of trust will result in insurmountable ramifications in attracting and maintaining donors, the very lifeblood of any charity. In the end, this means the death of the nonprofit, the very mission you wish to accomplish. We at FTS never really thought about this in the beginning. We were and continue to be brutally honest and accountable for any donation, no matter how big or small, but we never had a good grasp on HOW and what it meant to be accountable. As FTS grew and progressed into a business model, we realized the essential nature of translating this honesty and accountability into a real model for the public. We strive to demonstrate financial, moral, and outcomes accountability to our donors, who trust us to carry out our mission of helping children throughout the world.

With respect to fiscal accountability, FTS has annual audits by reputable nonprofit tax firms, submits timely form 990 forms, avoids any loans or payments to directors, and has a solid system of financial reporting, record keeping, and disclosure that allows others to examine our organization with ease. I will admit that this did not fall into place automatically. It was once again a learning process that took place over time. With all of the above in place, trust is portrayed to the public, and confidence is gained that you are a reputable charitable organization.

Moral accountability is essentially the role of the board of directors and executive director. The board members have the legal responsibility of upholding certain standards of conduct and responsibility to the organization and to the public. This one is hard to define in words, yet the very fabric of character and who you choose for your board play a large role in the moral accountability. Once again, I have learned just how important it is to properly define who will serve as your board of directors.

Outcomes accountability is one that FTS strives very hard to achieve. Being a cleft lip and palate foundation, we strive for perfection in our surgical repairs, much like we would here in the United States. Too often, untrained surgeons volunteer on these missions and operate on these impoverished children without experience. The results will almost always be subpar and result in the need for additional surgery in the future, which is always a losing battle because a secondary repair never can be as good as a well-done primary repair.

FTS achieves outcomes accountability by objectively evaluating surgeries performed, surgeons' abilities, and available infrastructure. Our standards of accountability are that we operate only in adequate facilities that hold to the same anesthetic standards as we do here in the United States. We will not provide anesthesia without appropriate monitors, inclusive of all the known standards in our very own hospitals at home. Oftentimes, this means transporting our own monitors, which can cost more money to the organization. If we perform cleft palate surgeries, we have to have access to an intensive care unit (ICU) and blood, were it to be necessary. If an ICU is not available, we will not perform the cleft palate repair. Again, this is just another standard of safety, accountability in a sense.

Postoperatively, we have adequate follow-up care provided for every patient to the best of our ability. It is tough for a cleft lip and palate charity doing surgery on an impoverished child who lives in the mountains 2 days journey away from the hospital to provide adequate follow-up for this child. In reality, it is almost impossible and may never happen as you wish it could. Postoperative care is oftentimes an outpost in or near their village, yet they always have access to our in-country host, who can get them to the proper hospital, if need be.

Finally, we try to get 3-week and 4-month postoperative photographs of our patients to assess our work. In truth, we may capture 50% of these photographs, but they are hugely helpful. FTS has collected nearly 200 postoperative photographs and keeps detailed records that document who the surgeon was, and when and where the surgery was performed. This record allows us to scrutinize each surgeon's work and better our missions. I have found this to be an invaluable tool in learning for myself and for others. Showing these photographs to donors, we are also able to demonstrate that we are accountable for our work. Granted, not every surgery is perfect or ideal, but FTS has confidence and evidence that our work is of good quality and that we truly are giving a great service to those children who so deserve to have a normal life.

FINAL PERSPECTIVE

Our mission experience has obviously had a dramatic effect on both of our lives. Without a doubt, we consider ourselves fortunate, the "lucky ones." Looking to the future, the exact fate of our mission work is to be determined but holds a large place in our lives and will continue to do so.

The true measure of greatness for any human being is how well he or she touches and treats another human being, especially for those who are less fortunate.

As FTS Foundation and A Smile for a Child Foundation continue to learn, grow, work, and expand, we only hope that we can continue to help many more in need.

A Smile for a Child Foundation and FTS Foundation are always in need of new donors to fulfill their mission. If you would like to contribute to either one of these foundations or have questions, please contact the authors. We would both like to acknowledge the hard work of our boards and volunteers as we cannot make this work without them.

A Smile for a Child Foundation:
1000 North Lincoln, Suite 2000
Oklahoma City, OK 73104
http://www.oklahomacleft.org/

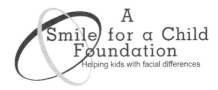

Free to Smile:
118 Graceland Boulevard, Suite 213
Columbus, OH 43214
http://www.freetosmile.org/

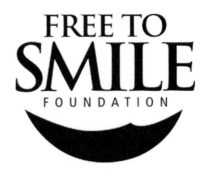

Index

Note: Page numbers of article titles are in **boldface** type.

Moving?

Make sure your subscription moves with you!

To notify us of your new address, find your **Clinics Account Number** (located on your mailing label above your name), and contact customer service at:

Email: journalscustomerservice-usa@elsevier.com

800-654-2452 (subscribers in the U.S. & Canada)
314-447-8871 (subscribers outside of the U.S. & Canada)

Fax number: 314-447-8029

Elsevier Health Sciences Division
Subscription Customer Service
3251 Riverport Lane
Maryland Heights, MO 63043

ELSEVIER

Printed and bound by CPI Group (UK) Ltd, Croydon, CR0 4YY

12/05/2025

01866863-0002